W9-DGP-466

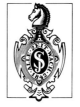

G. Hierholzer   Th. Rüedi
M. Allgöwer   J. Schatzker

Manual on the AO/ASIF Tubular External Fixator

With 104 Figures, Some in Colour

Springer-Verlag
Berlin Heidelberg New York Tokyo 1985

Professor Dr. med. Günther Hierholzer
Ärztlicher Direktor der Berufsgenossenschaftlichen
Unfallklinik Duisburg-Buchholz
Großenbaumer Allee 250
D-4100 Duisburg 28

Professor Dr. med. Thomas Rüedi
Chefarzt der Chirurgischen Klinik
Rätisches Kantons- und Regionalspital
CH-7000 Chur

Professor Dr. med. Martin Allgöwer
Präsident der AO International
Balderstraße 30
CH-3007 Bern

Joseph Schatzker, M.D. F.R.C.S. (C)
Associate Professor
110 Crescent Road
Toronto, Ontario, M4W 175
Canada

ISBN 3-540-13518-9 Springer-Verlag Berlin Heidelberg New York Tokyo
ISBN 0-387-13518-9 Springer-Verlag New York Heidelberg Berlin Tokyo

Library of Congress Cataloging in Publication Data

Fixateur-externe-osteosynthese. English. Manual on the AO/ASIF tubular external fixator.
   Translation of: Fixateur-externe-osteosynthese.
   Bibliography: p.
   Includes index.
   1. Fracture fixation-Handbooks, manuals, etc.
I. Hierholzer, G. (Günther), 1933–. II. Title.
III. Title: Manual on the A.O./A.S.I.F. tubular external fixator.
RD101.F5713   1985   617'.15   84-20196
ISBN 0-387-13518-9 (U.S.)

Typesetting, printing and bookbinding: Universitätsdruckerei H. Stürtz AG, D-8700 Würzburg
2124/3130-543210

Contents

1 Introduction and Basic Indications for the Use of External Skeletal Fixation

The history of external skeletal fixation begins in the middle of the 19th century with MALGAIGNE's [11] description of a simple unilateral frame. Since then considerable development has taken place. LAMBOTTE [10] pushed the development of the external fixator further and was the first to apply a simple unilateral frame in a systematic fashion. CODEVILLA [3] pioneered in describing the principles of the double-frame configuration, which was further developed by STADER [16] and HOFFMANN [6]. ANDERSON [1] described the half-pin "fracture units" with prestressing and recurrent compression of the fracture site. VIDAL and his co-workers [17] were the first to subject the various assemblies of the external fixator frames to mechanical testing. Their results were instrumental in gaining wider acceptance for this method. The external fixator was used in clinical practice to treat fractures and pseudarthroses, as well as in arthrodesis of the knee and ankle [13]. The advantages of this type of fixation – namely, fixation of the involved portion of the skeleton with sparing of the endangered soft and boue tissues – were recognized by the pioneers of external skeletal fixation.

The Association for the Study of Problems of Internal Fixation (AO) [5, 7–9, 12–15, 18] has also devoted itself to the problems of external skeletal fixation. Our early external fixation was characterized by the use of threaded bars in the assembly of the frames, which we applied – except in arthrodesis – without preload of the pins. Our clinical experience convinced us, however, that this type of external fixator frame did not provide sufficient versatility and stability for successful treatment of problem fractures, such as those with segmental bone loss or with a short metaphyseal fragment, or for treatment of the combination of instability and chronic osteitis. The introduction of the AO tubular system brought with it considerable improvements in the component parts [7, 15]. The greater stiffness of the tubes permitted bridging of greater distances with much more stability than with the early model. We will outline the principal features of the most important types of assemblies, as well as the indications for their use. Three basic indications for external skeletal fixation have specific biomechanical implications and should be considered separately:

1. Fresh fractures accompanied by severe soft tissue damage, particularly open fractures with second- or third-degree soft tissue injuries
2. Infected nonunion with badly compromised soft tissue cover
3. Corrective metaphyseal osteotomies and arthrodesis of various joints, mainly the knee and the ankle

In *freshly fractured cortical bone* of the diaphysis in long bones, even optimal biomechanical placement of the transfixing pins or Schanz screws may not permit sufficient stability for primary bone healing to take place. On the other hand, such fixation seems to be too rigid to exert a physiological stimulus for normal callus formation, because cases chosen for this technique have often had significant extra osseous soft tissue stripping. Externally fixed diaphyseal bone heals only slowly, or not at all, if no other surgical procedures are applied. Stabilization of fresh fractures by means of external skeletal fixation therefore has to take two other aspects into consideration. It must be clearly visualized as a means of coping with the soft tissue problem for the immediate post-trauma or postoperative period. When the soft tissue problem is under control, a second operative step, often such as bone grafting or even internal fixation, has to be considered. To carry out secondary internal fixation with maximum safety, the bone close to the fracture area should not be compromised by transfixing pins or screws. This results, of course, in a lesser degree of initial stability, because one must keep away from the fracture focus as much as possible. Another safety measure is to allow a 2–3 week interval between removal of the external fixator and the secondary procedure.

For fresh fractures there is one technique which can provide "absolute stability" in combination with external fixation: lag-screw fixation of the fracture plus neutralization by the external fixator.

In *infected nonunions*, where the soft tissue problems prevent the usual procedure of removing the dead bone in combination with cancellous bone transplant and internal fixation, we may have to rely on external fixation in conjunction with a cancellous autograft as a definitive means. In such cases we must strive for the reasonable optimum of mechanical stabilization by placing the Steinmann pins or Schanz screws in each main fragment at maximum distance from each other, thus coming close to the area of instability with the innermost pin or screw; in addition, we quite often use a three-dimensional frame, or an anterior and medial unilateral frame at a 60°–90° angle.

Where cancellous bone sections of the metaphysis are brought into contact in arthrodesis or osteotomy, compression fixation with an adequate two- or three-dimensional frame is so stable that very rapid bony union is achieved (8–12 weeks).

Under all three conditions it is most important to prevent loosening of pins and Schanz screws, which invariably leads to pin tract infection. Loosening is best prevented by putting the pins and Schanz screws under preload, by either *interfragmental compression* (across the focus of fracture) if bony support is warranted, e.g., in transverse fractures, osteotomies, or arthrodeses, or *intrafragmental compression* by prestressing the Steinmann pins and Schanz screws in cases with bony defects. Preload on the pins and Schanz screws is a most important ingredient of external fixation. Straight pins are under zero load and cause bone resorption and loosening due to micromovements. Adding a thread to Steinmann pins does not help much to prevent loosening; such pins are quite difficult to insert and remove, and should therefore be considered obsolete.

The main emphasis of this manual is on the application of the AO tubular system in fresh, open fractures of second and third degree; the other two indications are dealt with only briefly. The use of external skeletal fixation in pelvic and vertebral fractures is not covered here. Special indications are treated in the Appendix.

2 Mechanical Principles of External Skeletal Fixation

The point having been made that rigid stability is not the only, and often not even the main aim in using the external skeletal fixator, it is still important to explain the mechanics of its application and the relevance of application to stability.

The component parts of the tubular system allow various forms of assembly. We have tested the mechanical behavior of these assemblies and clinically defined their application. The horizontal and linear displacement of fragments were measured with strain gauges [7, 9] and the torsional stability was determined by means of "finite element analysis" [7]. The results obtained have led us to recognize three basic forms of assembly. We shall now discuss some of these mechanical features.

Once a fracture has been stabilized by an external fixator, the horizontal displacement of the fragments under load is used as one of the parameters for determining the achieved stability of fixation. Under eccentric load, which corresponds to the physiological conditions, we see that each main fragment is subject to a turning moment. This results in an almost exclusively horizontal displacement of the fragment ends. If we introduce one Steinmann pin in the frontal plane into the proximal fragment it becomes the centre of rotation of that fragment. If instead of one Steinmann pin we introduce two, the center of rotation is now found halfway between the two Steinmann pins. In the loaded system, the introduction of the second Steinmann pin causes a countermoment, which increases in magnitude as the distance between the two Steinmann pins increases. Thus, two pins are desirable because they give greater stability to the fragments in the horizontal plane. If one is dealing with a short metaphyseal fragment, and if it is impossible to introduce two Steinmann pins in the frontal plane, then the desired countermoment can be achieved by introducing a Schanz screw in a dorsoventral direction or in a sagittal plane. This considerably reduces the horizontal displacement of the fragments. The distance of the Schanz screw from the Steinmann pin which serves as the center of rotation should be as great as possible. This

5

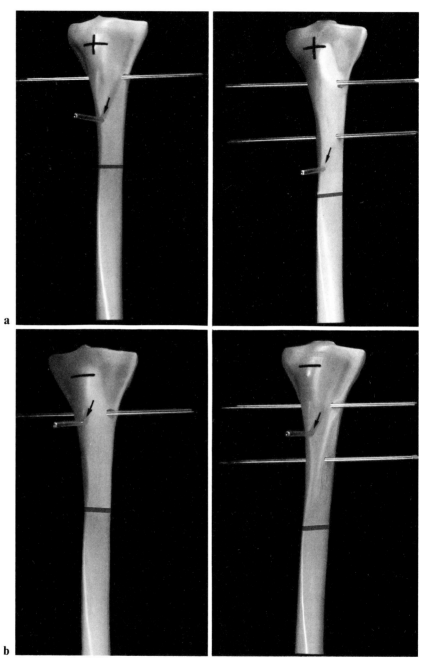

a

b

Fig.
1a, b
Insertion of two parallel Steinmann pins, or an additional Schanz screw in a dorsoventral direction. Decrease in horizontal displacement after production of a countermoment under eccentric load. **a** Correct position $(+)$ of the additionally inserted Schanz screw, as far from the center of rotation of the fragment as possible; **b** incorrect position $(-)$

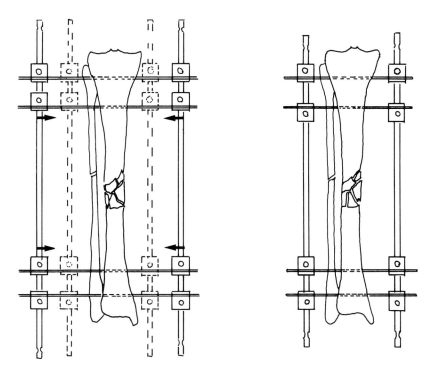

Fig. 2 Fixing the tubes as close to the limb as possible. Increase in the stability of the assembly with decrease in the free segment of the Steinmann pins and Schanz screws

means that the Schanz screw should be introduced as close to the fracture as is compatible with the overall treatment plan (Fig. 1 a).

The degree of horizontal displacement of the fragments can be further reduced by triangulation, in which a bilateral frame in the frontal plane is joined by means of oblique Steinmann pins with a unilateral frame which has been inserted ventrally in the sagittal plane. The stability is increased because the triangulation neutralizes both tensile and compressive forces. The triangulation also counteracts bending of the tubes. The stability of the system also depends on the free segments of the tubes, the Steinmann pins, and the Schanz screws, which can be subjected to bending and buckling. The shorter this segment for all component parts, the greater the stability and the lesser the displacement of the fragments. Therefore, if the external fixator is used to bridge long distances, the tube segment between the Steinmann pins adjacent to the fracture must be kept to an absolute minimum. Furthermore, the tubes should be fixed as close to the limb as possible in order to decrease the free distance of the Steinmann pins and of the Schanz screws (Fig. 2).

7

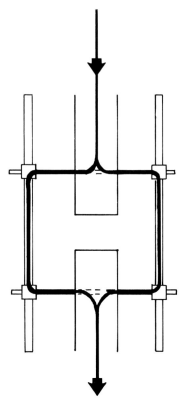

Fig. 3   When subjected to load, the direction of force in an assembly follows indicated path

One further important parameter used in the evaluation of the stability of an assembly is the linear or axial displacement of the fragments when subjected to load. The direction of force follows chiefly the path indicated in Fig. 3. The linear or axial displacement of an assembly is determined by the degree of bending of the Steinmann pins. This bending is in turn determined by the distance between the tubes, the diameter of the Steinmann pins, and their rigidity. The rigidity is dependent on the metal used. Our experiments have shown that preloading of the Steinmann pins by bending them towards one another can reduce the linear displacement of each main fragment by 45% (Fig. 4a, b). The horizontal displacement of the fragments is also reduced by preloading the pins, although to a much lesser degree, as was pointed out by ANDERSON [1] years ago. Preloading of the Steinmann pins in bone leads to a significant decrease in the

Fig. 4a, b   "Intrafragmentary" preloading of two Steinmann pins by bending them together in each main fragment. Reduction of the linear and horizontal displacement, as well as of metal loosening in bone

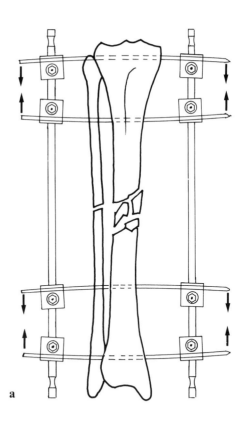

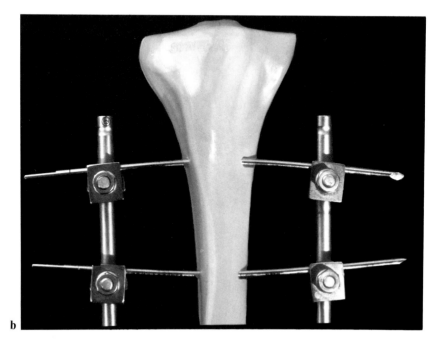

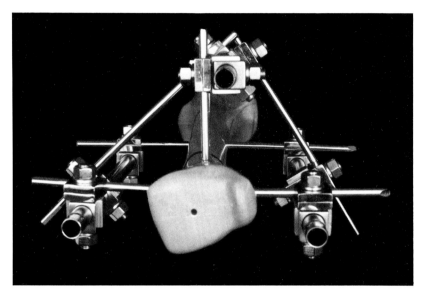

Fig. 5   Triangulated configuration of the assembly by linking the unilateral frame inserted in the sagittal plane to the bilateral frame inserted in the frontal plane, increasing rotational stability

incidence of loosening and to a considerable reduction in the danger of side slippage; it has made the use of threaded Steinmann pins obsolete.

In addition, the stability of an external fixator assembly is determined by its resistance to rotation or torsional moments. This is best measured by means of finite element analysis. Finite element calculations [7] have shown that a ventral tube can neutralize the torsional moments only in a three-dimensional configuration (Fig. 5). This means that the unilateral frame inserted in the sagittal plane must be linked to the bilateral frame inserted in the frontal plane. Triangulation leads principally to rotational stability. Its influence on the degree of horizontal displacement of the fragment is low.

The fixation of the tubes to the Steinmann pin results in a certain degree of eccentricity of the system. Because the load is applied eccentrically we must aim, when we lock the tubes in position, at minimizing the distance between the point of force application and the load axis. The reduction of this distance means the reduction of a lever arm which, if too long, could cause a bending of the tubes. The practical consequence of this is that in assembling the frame the side tubes should be fixed posterior or dorsal to the Steinmann pins (Fig. 6a, b).

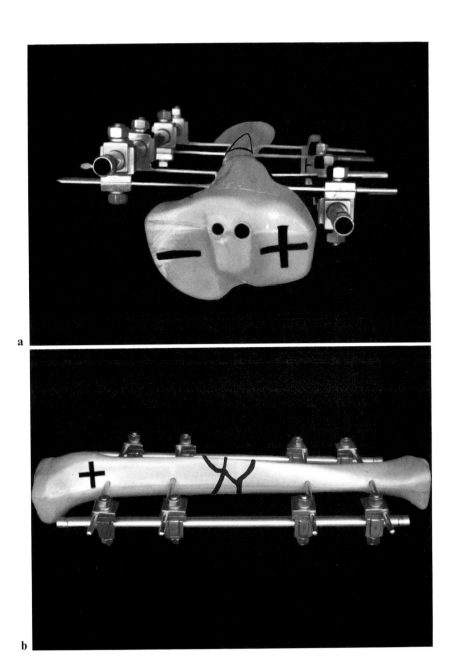

a

b

Fig.
6a, b
Fixation of the tubes dorsal to the Steinmann pins (+, correct; −, incorrect), showing reduction of the lever arm

3 Remarks Concerning the Pathophysiology of Compound Fractures

In animal experiments, an inoculum of pathogenic organisms on the order of $6–8 \times 10^6$ is required to create an abscess. In contrast, open fractures with considerable damage to the soft tissue and bone can be infected with a much smaller number of bacteria. The explanation for this lies, of course, in the fact that in damaged soft tissue and bone both cellular and humoral defense mechanisms have been seriously compromised.

Animal experiments, as well as clinical observations, provide ample proof that one should not undertake operative stabilization of problem fractures by internal fixation where complications such as infection and soft tissue necrosis are either impending or already established. The greater the soft tissue and bone damage, the greater the danger of infection.

As a rule, therefore, open fractures should be considered contaminated. If debridement of the wound has been delayed beyond the first 6–8 h after injury, the pathogenic organisms have passed through the lag phase and have entered the phase of multiplication. Under these circumstances an internal fixation with the associated implantation of a foreign body may bring with it a high risk of infection.

On the other hand, there is both experimental and clinical proof that immobilization of the area of injury is most important for the differentiation of pluripotential cells, a process which leads to revascularization. Hence, there are many arguments for operative stabilization of the fracture in order to enhance the local defense mechanisms and accelerate bone healing. The external fixator is thus an ideal device for the treatment of open fractures, especially of grades 2 and 3 with major soft tissue damage.

4 Indications for External Skeletal Fixation Versus Internal Fixation

If we limit ourselves in the use of the external fixator to its strictest indications, then it is not in competition with the standard procedures of internal fixation. The external fixator should be viewed rather as an alternative to the methods of intramedullary nailing or plating, applicable whenever nailing or plating is considered too hazardous. We must remember, however, that bony union of fresh fractures usually takes longer with external fixation than with rigid internal fixation. Exceptions, of course, are the osteotomies carried out in metaphyseal areas of bone, or joint arthrodesis, where broad surfaces of cancellous and well-vascularized bone are brought under compression. These considerations pertain more to the tibia than to other bones that are protected by more circumferential muscle cover, so that both a delay of internal fixation and the different devices are better tolerated.

The following are the indications for external skeletal fixation:

Diaphyseal and metaphyseal segment
1. Open grade-3 fractures
2. Open grade-2 fractures beyond 6–8 h after injury
3. Closed fractures with extensive soft tissue damage, contusions, or scar formation
4. Comminuted fractures in polytraumatized patients
5. Infected fractures and pseudarthroses
6. Corrective osteotomies

Articular segment (arthrodesis)
1. Post-traumatic osteoarthritis
2. Degenerative osteoarthritis
3. Septic arthritis

The surgical and clinical advantages of stabilization with the external fixator can be summarized as follows:

15

Surgical characteristics of external skeletal fixation

- Stability without interfering with the endangered fracture area
- Stability despite a bony defect
- The possibility for primary or secondary bone grafting
- The possibility of conversion to another type of fixation

Clinical characteristics of external skeletal fixation

- Ease of wound care
- Ease of postoperative positioning of the patient
- Possibility of mobilization of adjacent joints
- Shortening of hospital stay

5 Four Building Components of the AO Tubular System and the Accompanying Surgical Instruments

Most external fixation systems are rather complex. They do not achieve stability between bone and pins by preload, and they do not make use of optimal stability of the connecting rods. Furthermore, they try to replace preoperative planning and thinking by making extreme external and rotational corrections possible after application of the external fixator. In contrast, the AO/ASIF external fixator was conceived to combine stability and versatility, making use of only four basic elements: *Simplicity is the rule of the game* (Fig. 7).

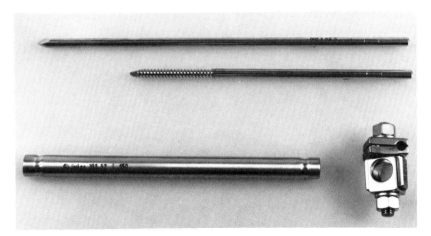

Fig. 7   Four basic building components

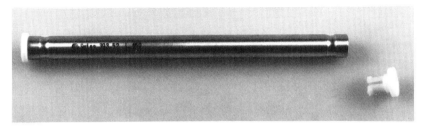

Fig. 8   Tube, and tube caps

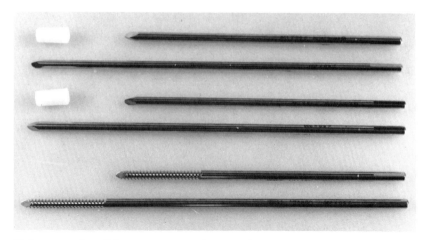

Fig. 9 Steinmann pins, Schanz screws, and protective caps

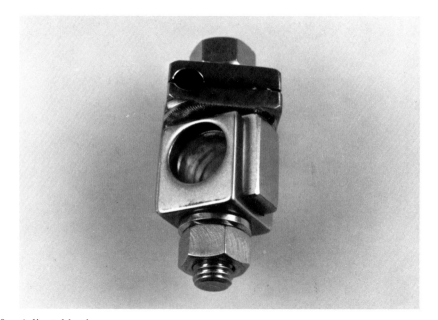

Fig. 10 Adjustable clamp

Fig. 11 a–c Versatility of the adjustable clamp which connects Steinmann pins, tubes, and Schanz screws

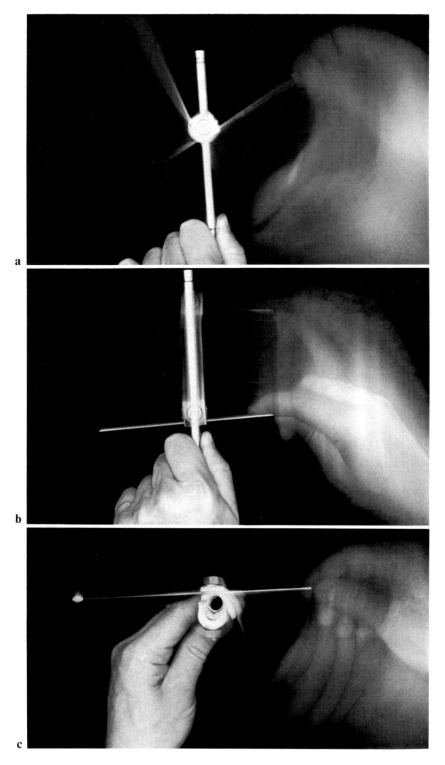

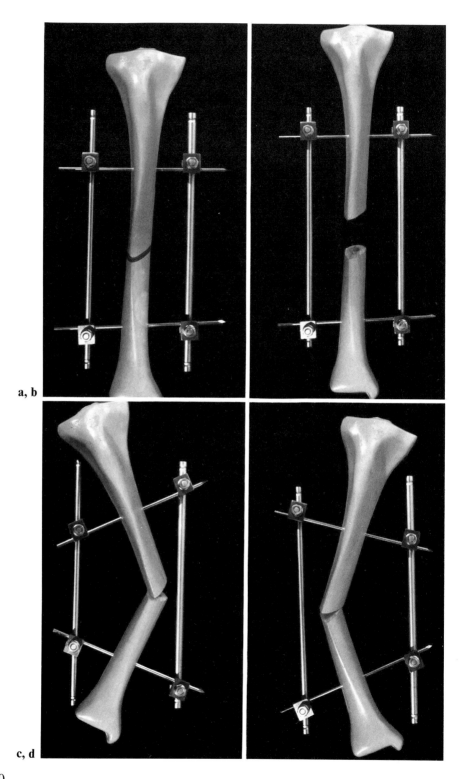

a, b

c, d

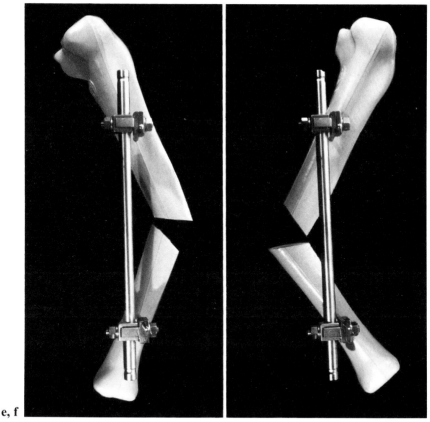

e, f

Fig.
12a–f The adjustable clamp makes it possible to correct the axis in all planes after the external fixator has been assembled. Correction of (**a, b**) a linear displacement, (**c, d**) a varus or valgus displacement, (**e, f**) a backward or forward displacement

The first building block (Fig. 8) is the tube, which comes in various lengths (100–600 mm) and has an outer diameter of 11 mm. The tube is roughly two-and-a-half times as rigid as the earlier threaded bar. It is therefore much more suitable for bridging long distances. In addition, the use of the tube has greatly simplified the fixation and removal of the adjustable clamps.

The second building block is the 5-mm Steinmann pin, which comes in lengths ranging from 150 to 250 mm; the third is the Schanz screw, 5 mm in diameter, which comes in lengths varying from 100 to 200 mm (Fig. 9; see also Addendum).

The fourth and most useful building block (Fig. 10) is the adjustable clamp, which makes it possible to connect the other three

21

components. The adjustability of the clamp allows for corrections in all planes (Figs. 11–13). This feature permits completion of a reduction, or correction of a poor reduction not recognized at the time of surgery. With these four building blocks we are able to construct all the important assemblies of the external fixator. Other components which some authors recommend and use are available on request; in principle, we recommend that one restricts oneself to the four basic building blocks.

The fact that only four components are necessary for the construction of any frame is the essential beauty of the system, making both inventory and use extremely simple without sacrificing versatility.

A foot plate with its corresponding connecting piece is useful in the prevention of postoperative equinus (Fig. 14). Also available are special plastic protectors to cover the sharp tips of the Steinmann pins, as well as plastic plugs to insert into the holes of the tubes. These are supplementary items which have absolutely no bearing on the assembly of an external fixator; therefore, we do not consider them basic components.

For fixation with the AO tubular fixator the following instruments are necessary (Fig. 15): 3.5- and 4.5-mm drill bits; a 3.5-mm trocar, or a 5-mm Steinmann pin serving as a trocar; drill sleeves with inner diameters of 3.5 and 5.0 mm; a hand chuck for the insertion of Schanz screws and Steinmann pins; a compressor for compression or distraction. The aiming device is most useful if a frame is applied; it seats the drills, and consequently the Steinmann pin, in such a way that they meet the opposing adjustable clamp precisely. For tightening the nuts an open-end wrench or a socket wrench is used.

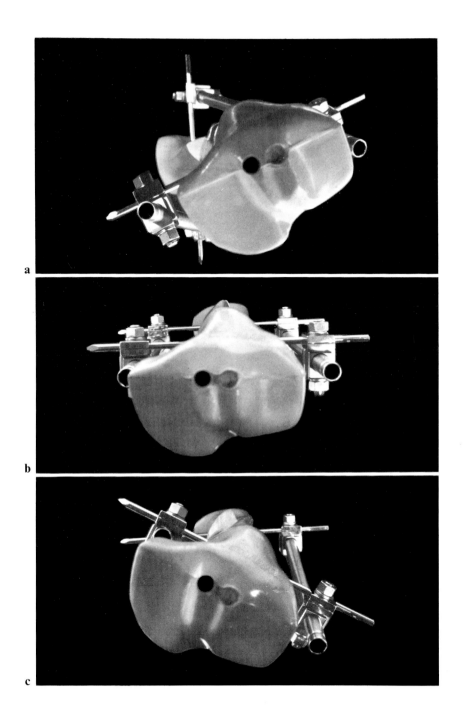

Fig.
13a–c   Correction of a rotational displacement with the adjustable clamp

23

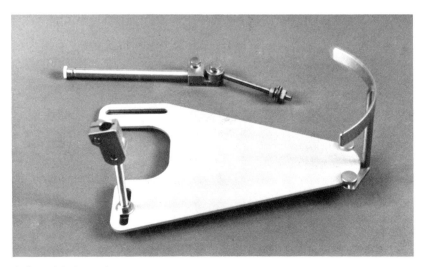

Fig. 14   Adjustable foot plate

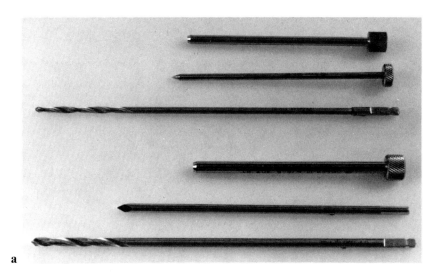

a

Fig.   Accessories to the external fixator. **a** Top to bottom: 3.5 mm drill sleeve;
15a–d   3.5 mm trocar; 3.5 mm drill bit, extra long; 5.0 mm drill sleeve; 5.0 mm
Steinmann pin (serving as trocar); 4.5 mm drill bit, extra long. **b–d** Hand
chuck

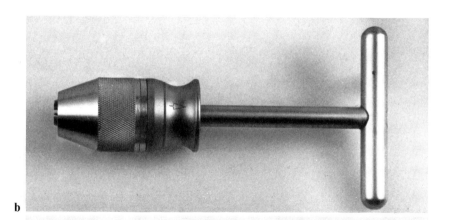

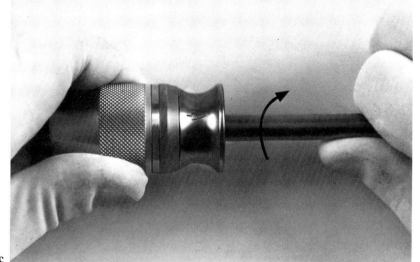

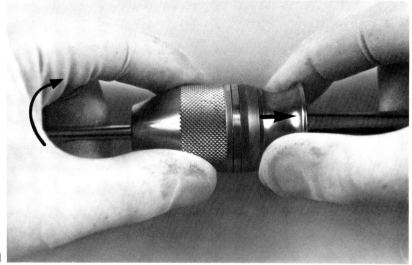

25

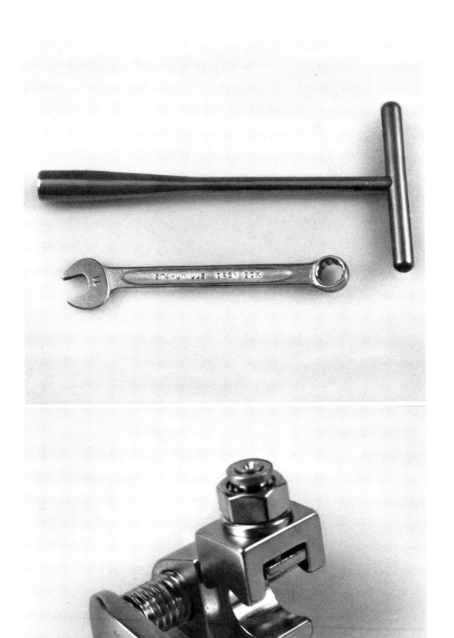

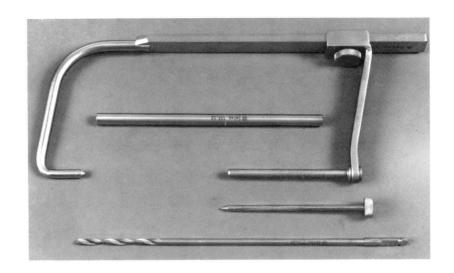

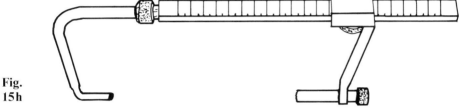

Fig. 15 **e** Socket wrench (11 mm) and open-end wrench (11 mm). **f** Compressor. **g, h** Aiming device

27

6 Basic Assemblies and Their Use

Many forms of assembly are possible with the previously described building blocks. However, we wish to single out three basic types. They are represented schematically in Fig. 16. Our experiments have shown that each of these basic assemblies is characterized by different mechanical properties. If one considers the topographical and anatomical features of an injury, one will recognize that all three forms of assembly have their application. In the description which follows we have not attempted to represent a systematic classification of the system with indications for its use. It should become clear to the reader that the surgeon must consider the clinical as well as the mechanical problems which an injury presents before deciding on the most suitable assembly of the external fixator. Therefore, the following presentations are not meant as a rigid scheme for the application of the external fixator but rather as a general guide.

Unilateral Frame, Type I

The type-I assembly (Figs. 17–20), is best suited for the stabilization of regions where the local topography and anatomy and functional considerations make the erection of a double frame or of a triangulated assembly inadvisable or impossible. For the upper extremity the unilateral one-plane frame external fixator must be used almost exclusively, e.g., for the humeral shaft, ulna, and radius, and occasionally for stabilization of comminuted fractures of the distal radius. For the upper extremities, the stability achieved with the unilateral frame is usually sufficient. Furthermore, this type of assembly allows the surgeon to pay greater attention to the course of important nerves and vessels. It also allows for early mobilization of the adjacent joints.

If there is a clinical indication for external fixation in open fractures of the femur, the unilateral one-plane frame is the one most frequently used. An exception to this rule are fractures of the distal femur. The stability of a unilateral one-plane frame external fixator is considerably lower, however, than that achieved by means of internal fixation. Thus, in the femur, the use of the external fixator should be restricted to the treatment of third-degree open fractures with extensive comminution, to the treatment of chronic osteitis or nonunion, and to femoral lengthening [4].

The unilateral frame in the sagittal plane assembly for fractures of the tibia, as advocated by BEHRENS and SEARLS [2], has recently become very popular. The advantages of this type of external fixator in the sagittal plane are that the anterolateral muscle compartment is not penetrated by multiple pins, and that it is well suited to neutralizing most of the bending forces which tend to cause displacement of the fragments. We feel that the unilateral frame is suited for the tibia, provided that it is not meant to be the definitive form of treatment and that, once healing of the associated soft tissue injuries has taken place, a conversion to internal fixation or functional cast bracing with or without bone grafting is considered. The choice of the type of external fixator used and the subsequent placement of the pins is therefore governed by the plan for the whole course of treatment and not only by temporary considerations. A V-shaped, or two-plane unilateral frame increases stability for long-range planning (Fig. 20) and can be made even more stable by linking the two bars together.

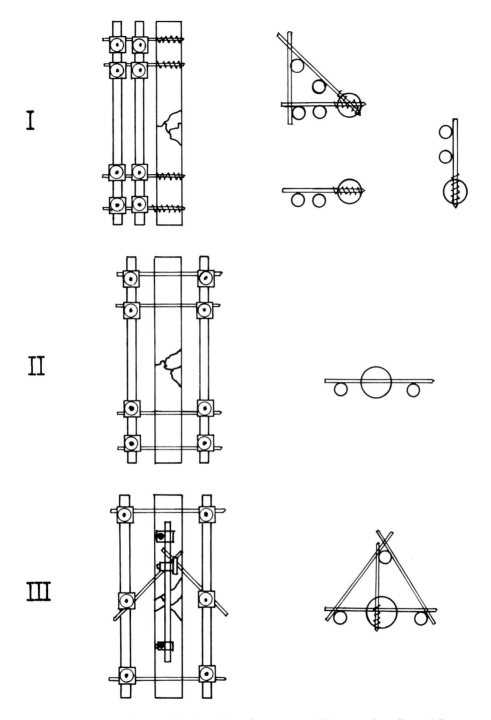

Fig. 16 Three basic forms of AO tubular fixator assembly: type I, unilateral form, one-plane, two-planes (V-shaped); type II, bilateral frame; type III, triangulated assembly

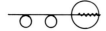

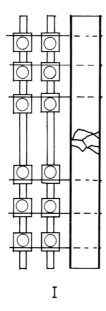

I

Fig. 17 Unilateral frame (type I) with one or two tubes

**Fig.
18 a–d** Unilateral frame (type I), on the radius (**a, b**) and on the femur (**c, d**)

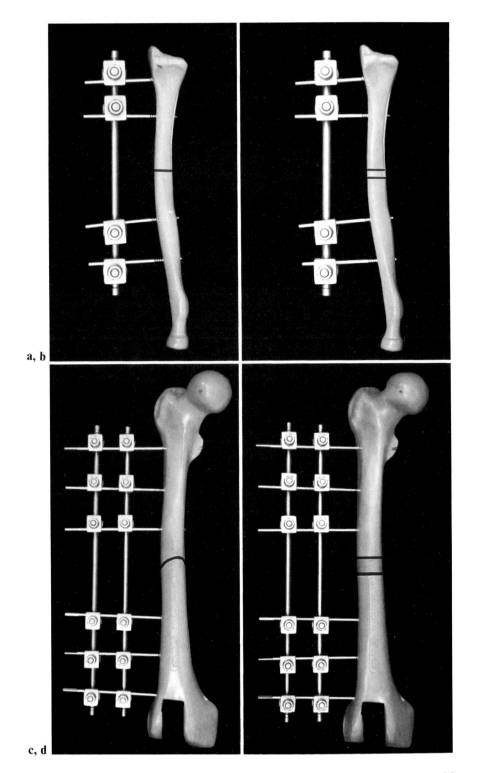

a, b

c, d

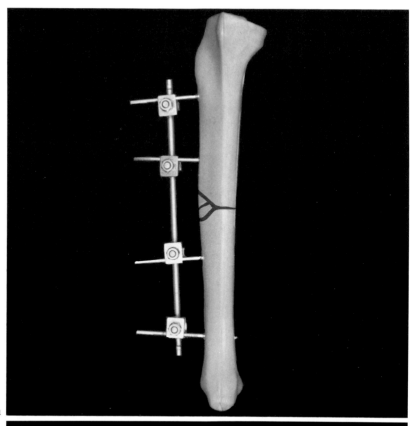

a

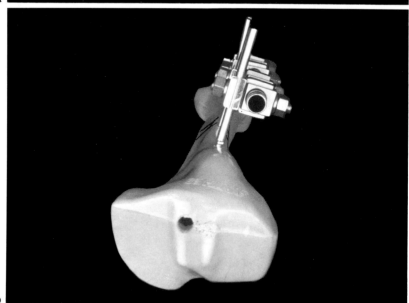

19 a, b   Unilateral frame (type I) in the ventrodorsal direction on the tibia

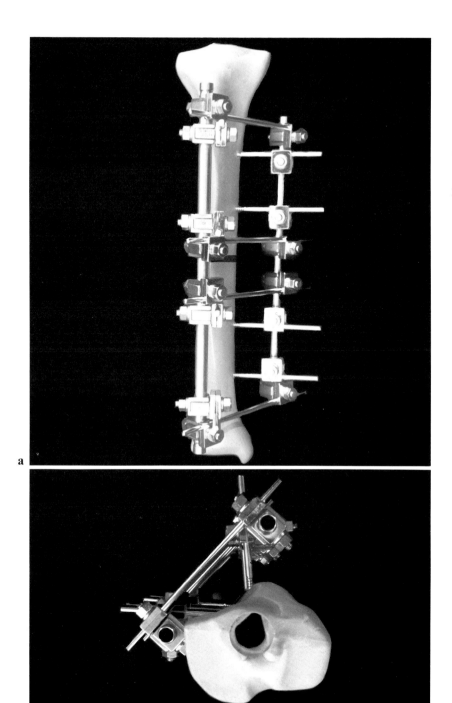

a

b

Fig.
20 a, b   V-shaped, or two-plane unilateral frame (type I) on the tibia

Bilateral Frame, Type II

The bilateral frame (Fig. 21) finds its chief application in fractures of the tibia. The stability of the bilateral frame assembly can be considerably increased by the already described principle of an additional lag screw and by preloading of the Steinmann pins. There are basically two ways in which this frame is applied, depending on whether there is bone contact or bone loss.

Condition 1: Bone Contact. If there is sufficient bone contact, as for instance in a transverse or short oblique fracture or in the case of an osteotomy, axial compression can be employed. This means that the Steinmann pins of the proximal and distal fragment are preloaded, or bent toward the fracture or osteotomy (Fig. 22a).

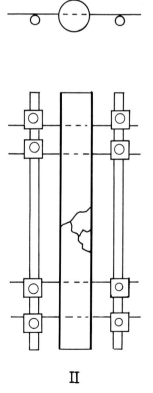

II

Fig. 21 Bilateral frame (type II)

If the fracture to be stabilized is oblique or spiral and has a tendency to slide, it is best to first achieve interfragmentary compression using one or two lag screws (Fig. 23). Depending on the stability produced by the lag screws, the bilateral frame is either applied with axial compression or used simply to neutralize bending and shearing forces. If axial compression is to be applied, the lag screw should be inserted at a right angle to the long axis of the bone.

Condition 2: Bone Defect. This condition is characterized by two situations: Either the area to be stabilized shows bone loss or severe comminution, or there is a defect and a chronic infection as well. Under these circumstances we cannot apply axial compression unless we are prepared to accept shortening. Thus, whenever there is a bony defect the external fixator has the task not only of maintaining length but also of acting as neutralizing device. Our experiments have shown that in the presence of a bony defect both axial and lateral displacement can be minimized by preloading the Steinmann pins within each main fragment (Fig. 22b). This increases the stability of the whole assembly and greatly improves the fit of the Steinmann pins in bone, thus preventing lateral slipping, loosening, and pin tract irritation or sepsis.

These two variations, i.e., either axial compression or the preloading of the Steinmann pins against one another in each of the two main fragments, have made the use of threaded pins generally unnecessary.

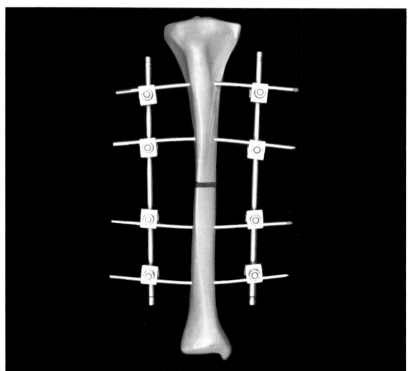

a

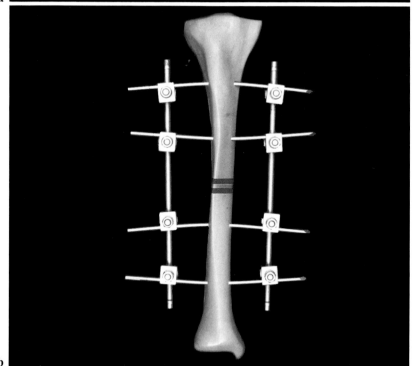

b

38

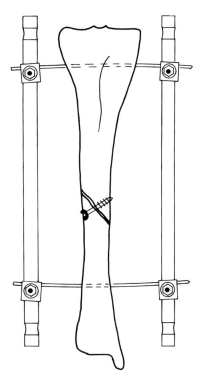

Fig. 23   Bilateral frame (type II) and additional interfragmentary compression by a lag screw in an oblique fracture of the tibia. In this case the bilateral frame is used to neutralize the bending and shearing forces

Fig.   Bilateral frame (type II) on the tibia. **a** *Inter*fragmentary compression with
22 a, b   bone contact. **b** Preloading of Steinmann pins within each fragment (*intra-*
               fragmentary compression) in the case of bone defect

Triangulated Assembly, Type III

Triangulated assembly (Figs. 24–27) is indicated mainly in the tibia, occasionally in the distal femur, and very rarely in the region of the elbow. The three-dimensional assembly is an alternative to the bilateral or V-shaped frame. The axial and lateral stability achieved with type-II and type-III configurations is about the same. The advantage of triangulated fixation, however, consists in its greater torsional stability, and in the fact that it is achieved with fewer anchoring pieces in bone. Thus, use of the triangulated type-III assembly can considerably reduce the number of Steinmann pins needed to transfix the lateral muscular compartment. The Schanz screws inserted in a sagittal plane into the anterior crest of the tibia almost never cause any irritation of the adjacent soft tissue or skin.

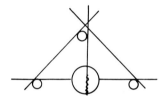

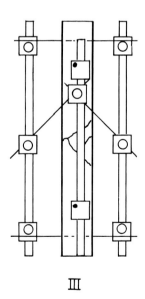

Fig. 24 Triangulated assembly of the external fixator (type III)

The principles of use already discussed for the bilateral frame also apply to the triangulated assembly. Thus, in the presence of bony contact we resort to axial compression. If, on the other hand, there is a large bony defect, we can achieve the greatest degree of stability by combining triangulated fixation with pre-loading of the two Steinmann pins in each main fragment. This type of assembly is particularly suited if long-term external fixation is reguired – for instance, in the treatment of chronic osteitis with bone loss.

The triangulated assembly is also very useful for arthrodesis of the knee and of the elbow. The ventral unilateral frame is linked with the bilateral frame by means of oblique Steinmann pins (Fig. 27). This type of configuration neutralizes the bending moments in the ventrodorsal or sagittal plane, which is of great advantage in the postoperative mobilization of the lower extremity after arthrodesis of the knee joint.

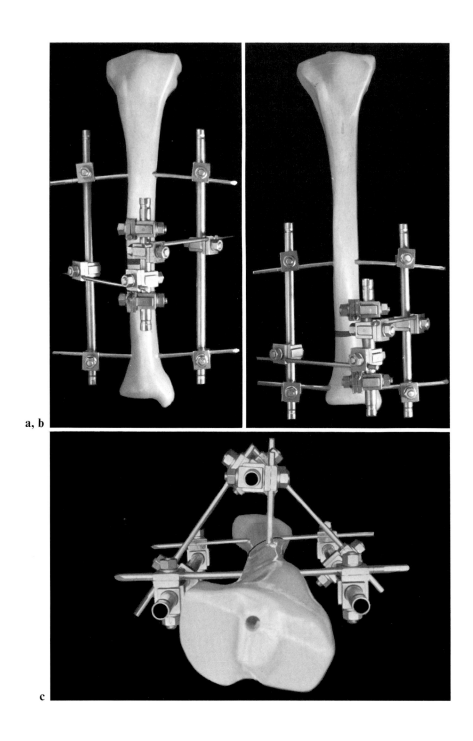

Fig. 25 a–c Triangulated assembly (type III). Diaphyseal (**a**) and metaphyseal (**b**) fractures with bone contact which allows axial compression. **c** Axial view

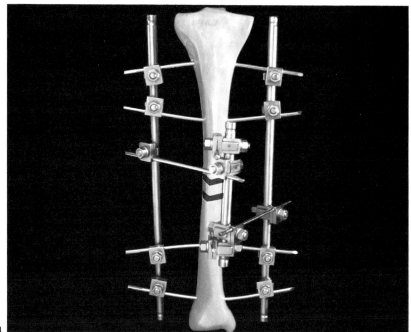

a

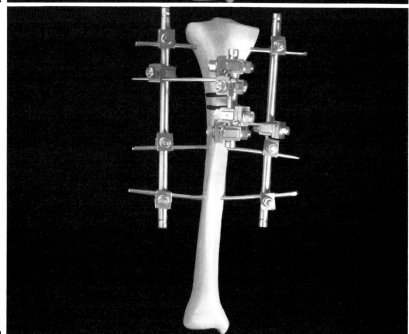

b

Fig.
26a, b
Triangulated assembly (type III). Diaphyseal (**a**) and metaphyseal (**b**) fractures with bone defect. Preloading of the Steinmann pins in each main fragment

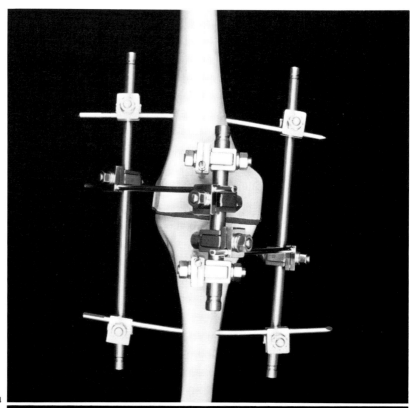

a

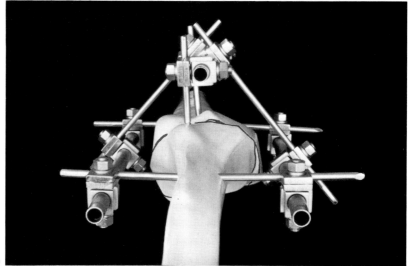

b

Fig. Triangulated assembly, (type III) for arthrodesis of the knee joint. **a, b**
27a, b Axial compression by the bilateral frame, triangulation for neutralization
of the bending moment in the sagittal plane

44

7 Technical Details for Construction

We shall now describe in detail all the steps necessary for the assembly of the external fixator frames with the four building components of the AO tubular system. We shall begin with the tibia, because the external fixator is most frequently used for stabilization of this bone.

One- and Two-plane Unilateral Frame (Type I) on the Tibia

With only slight modifications we follow the procedure advocated by BEHRENS and SEARLS [2]. Using the solid cortex of the anterior tibial crest is becoming more and more popular, as it offers the best "tension-band arrangement" and allows the tube to be very close to the bone. Axial and rotational alignment should be obtained first. One Schanz screw is inserted into each main fragment by means of a small stab incision close to the joint of each fragment, and a 3.5-mm hole is made, using a drill guide to protect the soft tissues. Care should be taken to place the screw within the sector of safe pin insertion (avoiding the muscular compartment) by means of the hand chuck, in a location where it will interfere as little as possible with debridement and secondary procedures (Fig. 28 a, b). Because of the risk of heat generation and bone necrosis the power drill must not be used for screw insertion. When a hole is drilled in the tibial head, close to the joint, the knee should be flexed so that the popliteal or tibial arteries are not hit.

A tube of appropriate length is selected and four (to six) adjustable clamps are mounted. The most proximal clamp and the most distal clamp are then connected to the first two Schanz screws (Fig. 28 c). After slight distraction of the fracture fragments a manual reduction is effected. Tightening of the most proximal and distal clamps secures the reduction temporarily and makes the insertion of subsequent screws easier. As malrotation is difficult to correct once all four pins are in place, particu-

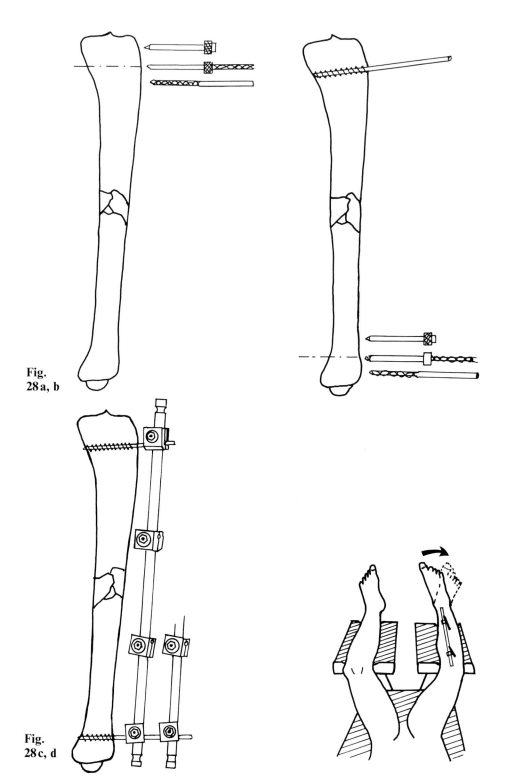

Fig. 28 a, b

Fig. 28 c, d

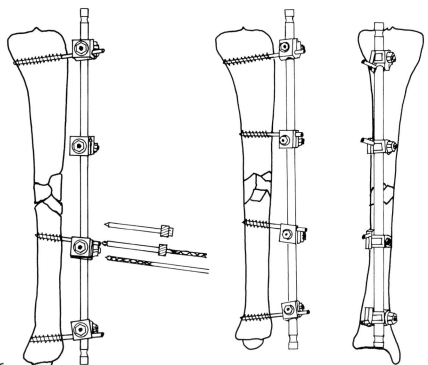

Fig.
28 e, f

lar attention must be directed to proper rotational alignment of the main fracture fragments before subsequent drilling (Fig. 28 d). One should attempt to get a perfect anatomic reduction at this time; sometimes an interfragmentary lag screw may be necessary.

Through the remaining clamps on the tube the other pin sites are predrilled, using a 3.5-mm drill bit, and the other Schanz screws are inserted with the hand chuck (Fig. 28 e, f). The drill sleeve protects the soft tissue and acts as a guide for drilling. The clamp screw must not be tightened too much when the sleeve is inserted through the clamp, as tightening may damage the thin sleeve wall.

If the addition of a second tube is planned, this second tube must be brought into the place before the third and fourth Schanz screws are inserted. (Fig. 28 c, g) [4]. In areas of broader bone contact axial compression can be applied (*inter*fragmental compression). This is not possible with bone defect, however, as the length of the limb should be saved. In such cases, preloading of the Schanz screws in each main fragment (*intra*fragmental compression) will avoid loosening of the screws.

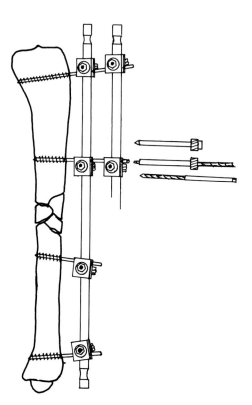

Fig.
28 g

If a two-plane or V-shaped unilateral fixation is desired, a second frame is mounted within the "sector of safe pin insertion" at a 60°–90° angle to the initially placed sagittal unilateral frame. Such an arrangement offers better rotational stability and markedly increased rigidity, and may be constructed as shown in Fig. 20. Should the necessity of axial correction arise, a hinge connector can be used between two appropriate rods.

Bilateral Frame (Type II) on the Tibia

Begin distally on the lateral side just above the ankle, and choose the point where you wish to insert the Steinmann pin. This should be anterior to the fibula. Make a stab incision and introduce the 3.5-mm trocar together with its corresponding drill sleeve down to the bone. It should be inserted at 90° to the long axis and parallel to the axis of the ankle joint. Remove the trocar from the drill sleeve which serves as the soft tissue protector and as a guide. With the 3.5-mm bit drill the first hole in the tibia. The hardness of the bone will indicate whether the hole needs to be enlarged or not. If the cortex feels very hard, the 3.5-mm hole should be enlarged with the 4.5-mm drill. In osteoporotic bone and in most metaphyseal areas a 3.5-mm hole is large enough for a 5.0-mm Steinmann pin and does not require enlargement.

With the aid of the hand chuck insert the first Steinmann pin (diameter 5 mm, length 180 mm) through the predrilled hole (Fig. 29a). Insertion with the hand chuck may be quite difficult. Once the pin passes through the medial cortex it is possible to complete its insertion using a hammer. A power drill should never be used for the insertion of Steinmann pins or Schanz screws, as considerable heat is generated, which usually leads to bone necrosis and formation of a sequestrum.

At the proximal tibia, proceed in a similar fashion. The stab incision is again placed anterior to the fibula, and the trocar with the corresponding drill sleeve is inserted down to the lateral cortex of the tibia. Before the proximal pin track is drilled, an attempt should be made to realign the leg and reduce the fracture as well as possible. This maneuver does not complicate the construction of the frame, but results in a much better positioning of the Steinmann pin without twisting of the tubes. It is quite difficult to determine the knee-joint axis in the presence of an unstable tibial fracture. By applying traction to the foot a preliminary reduction of the fracture is obtained and axial and rotational alignment of the tibia may also be controlled. Now place the proximal drill sleeve parallel to the distal Steinmann pin and drill a 3.5-mm hole through both cortices of the tibia. If the bone is very hard, enlarge the hole to 4.5 mm (Fig. 29b). Insert the second Steinmann pin (5 mm in diameter, 180 mm in length) through this hole with a hand chuck and a hammer, as already described (Fig. 29c).

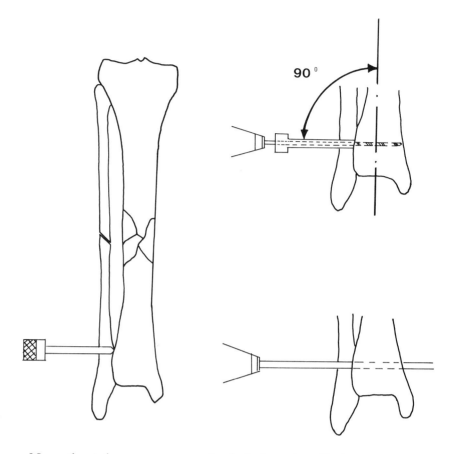

90°

Fig.
29 a

Now the tubes are prepared; their length will depend on the distance to be bridged. The number of adjustable clamps will depend on the type of assembly to be erected. Slip the adjustable clamps onto the tubes in such a way that their broad part comes to lie anterior to the Steinmann pins, the tube posterior to them. This will minimize the distance between the line of force and load application. If the lever is kept as short as possible the bending moment of the tubes is reduced as well. Once the simple frame is erected, turn the nuts slightly (Fig. 29d–f).

Now check the reduction once again, with particular regard to rotation of the fragments. In case of a poor alignment any correction must be done before the adjustable clamps are fully tightened. The fracture is now sufficiently stabilized to permit further manipulation and the insertion of the remaining pins (Fig. 29g, h).

For the insertion of the remaining pins we prefer to use the aiming device, as it almost guarantees that the additional Stein- mann pins will point in the right direction to go through the

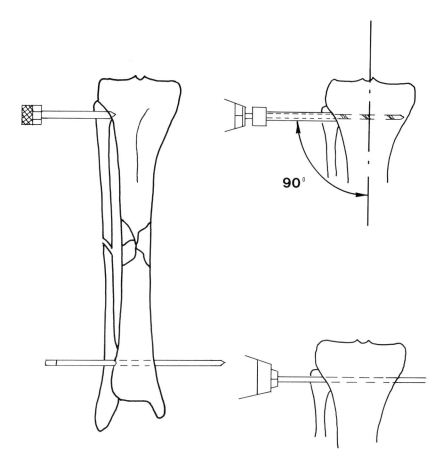

Fig.
29 b

adjustable clamps on the other side of the bone. At a suitable distance from the first Steinmann pin and sufficently removed from either the fracture or the focus of infection place the third and fourth stab incisions anterior to the fibula. The aiming device is then hooked into the lateral as well as the medial adjustable clamp, and the drill sleeve with trocar is pushed through the aiming device until it makes contact with the lateral cortex of the tibia (Fig. 29i). In order to guarantee the position tighten both adjustable clamps slightly; remove the trocar and proceed to drill the holes as already described.

The aiming device is now removed and the third and fourth Steinmann pins are introduced with the hand chuck. The Steinmann pins do not need to be precisely parallel to one another in the frontal plane, because the adjustable clamps allow for some degree of correction.

The distance of the Steinmann pins from the area of injury is determined (a) by the degree of soft tissue damage and (b) by

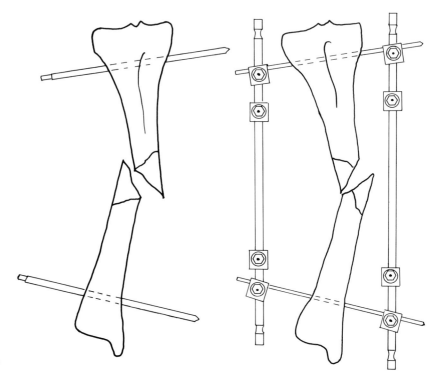

**Fig.
29 c, d**

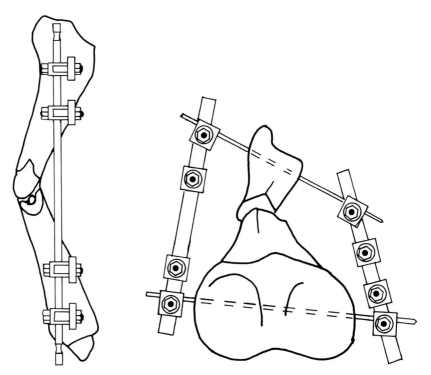

**Fig.
29 e, f**

52

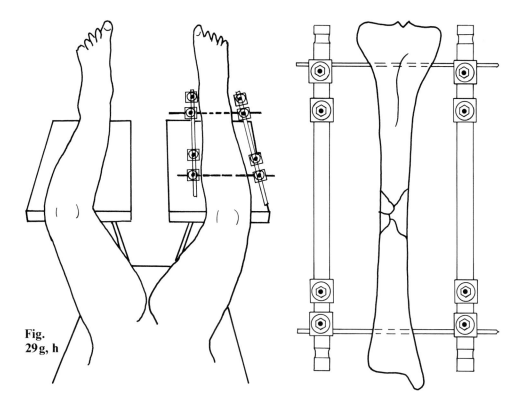

Fig.
29 g, h

the decision on whether the external fixator will be a definitve means of fixation or a further procedure is planned for the near future. For mechanical reasons, the closer the Steinmann pins are to the fracture site, the greater is the stability of the assembly. However, if internal fixation as a second step is anticipated, the pins should be kept as far away from the fracture area as possible, in order not to interfere with a future plate fixation. The tubes are placed as close to the skin as possible, keeping the distance between bone and tubes at a minimum. This also reduces their bending and buckling.

If a *fracture with a bone loss* has to be stabilized, it is desirable to increase the stability of the assembly to a maximum (Fig. 29j, k). This can be achieved by preloading the Steinmann pins within each main fragment against one another. Once they are bent towards one another the adjustable clamps are tightened. The preloading of the Steinmann pins must be done synchronously in each of the main fragments, otherwise one ends up with distraction or even angulation of the fracture.

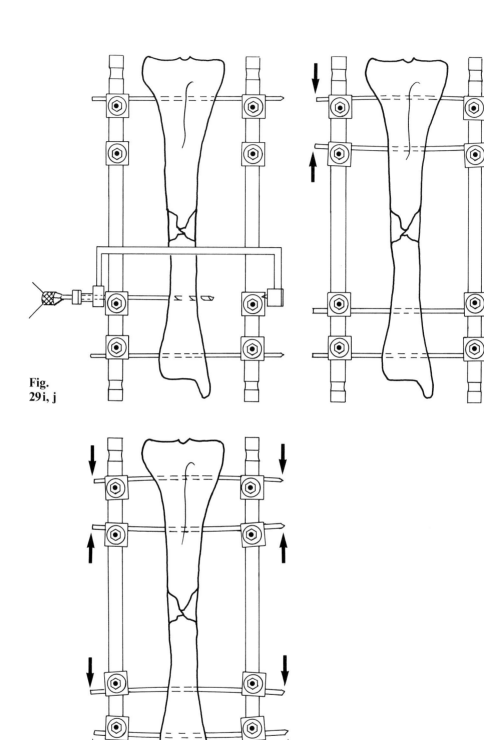

Fig. 29 i, j

Fig. 29 k

Oblique fractures should first be reduced and stabilized by lag screws. In this case, the external fixator acts as a neutralizing frame (Fig. 30a–g).

In case of a *transverse or very short oblique fracture* the stability is increased by axial compression (Fig. 30h, i). To achieve this, each pair of Steinmann pins is approximated towards the fracture and is fixed in this position. This "bending" of the Steinmann pins can be done by fixing a compressor into the tubes, by means of a Verbrugge clamp, or simply by hand. During preloading of the Steinmann pins, of course, both nuts of the corresponding adjustable clamps must be loosened. (Fig. 30e–g).

At the end of the operation care must be taken that the skin is not stretched at the exit points of the Steinmann pins. The incision should be widened at the point of tension, and a suture added on the opposite side. If the skin is under tension, this invariably leads to local irritation and possibly to pin tract infection.

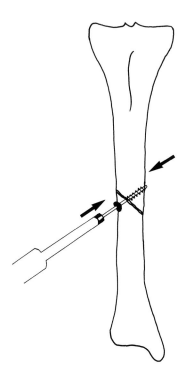

**Fig.
30 a**

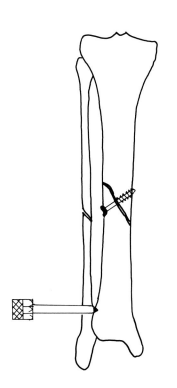

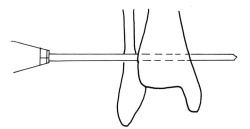

90⁰

**Fig.
30 b**

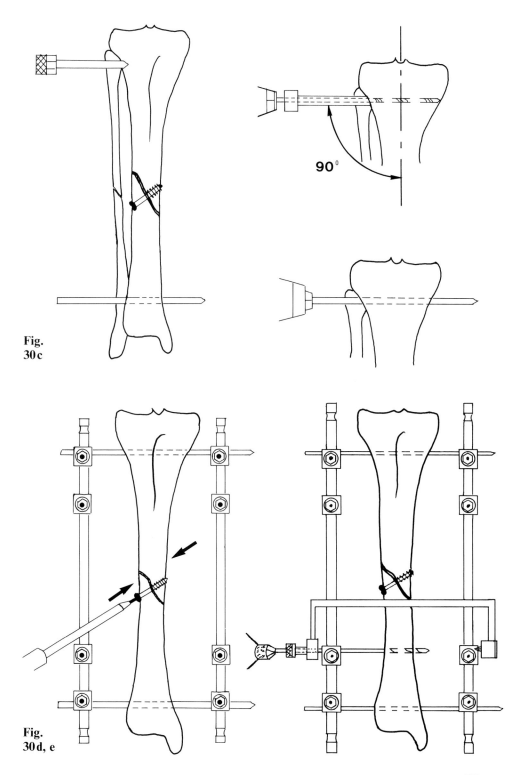

Fig.
30 c

90⁰

Fig.
30 d, e

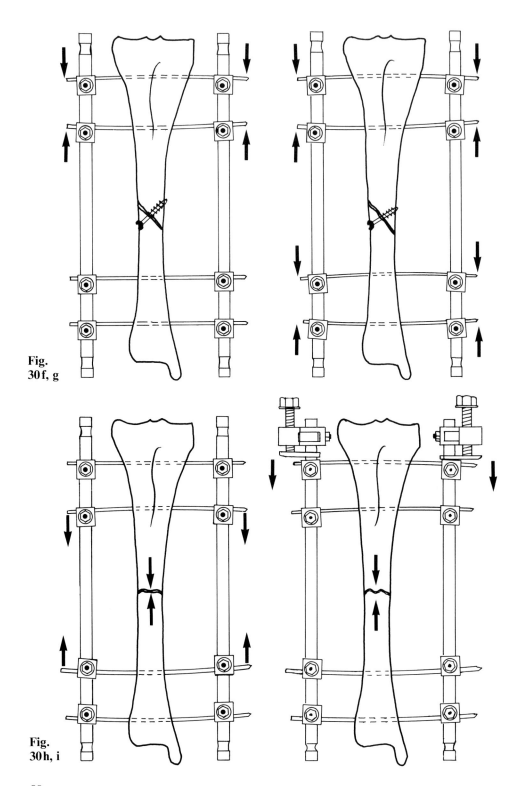

**Fig.
30 f, g**

**Fig.
30 h, i**

58

Triangulated Assembly (Type III) on the Tibia

As already described for the bilateral frame, one Steinmann pin in the frontal plane is inserted into the proximal and distal fragments. Three adjustable clamps are slipped into each of the side tubes, and a simple bilateral frame is constructed. The fracture is reduced under traction and the adjustable clamps are tightened. After the quality of reduction has been checked one Schanz screw is inserted in the sagittal plane into each of the main fragments. Care must be taken not to penetrate the posterior structures excessively with the tip of the Schanz screw, which is inserted with the hand chuck.

A third tube is prepared with four adjustable clamps. Two of the clamps are used to fix the tube to the Schanz screws, the other two to connect the ventral tube by means of oblique Steinmann pins to the bilateral frame. This completes the assembly of the triangulated frame (Fig. 31). Here, too, it is mandatory either to apply axial compression or to preload the Steinmann pins in pairs as already described (Fig. 32).

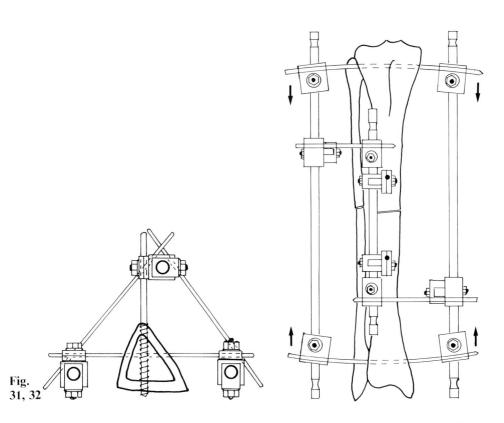

Fig. 31, 32

59

If we have to bridge a bony defect, the bilateral frame with the preloaded Steinmann pins limits axial and lateral displacement at the fracture site. The triangulation adds to rotational and torsional stability (Fig. 33). While erecting these assemblies it is important to make certain that the Schanz screws are not inserted into the axis of rotation of the paired Steinmann pins (see p. 6, Fig. 1). The Schanz screw is mechanically effective only if it is inserted at a distance from the axis of rotation of the paired Steinmann pins. The greater this distance, the more effective the fixation of the additional Schanz screw.

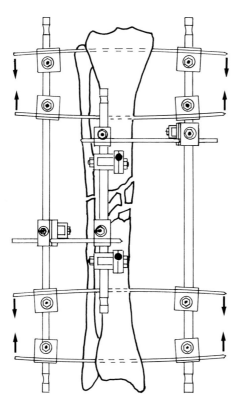

Fig. 33

Construction of a Unilateral Single-plane Fixator
(Type I) on the Femur Using Two Parallel Unilateral Tubes

Make a stab incision on the lateral side of the thigh and insert the trocar with its corresponding drill sleeve down to the femur, the drill sleeve acting as a tissue protector. In the frontal plane, a 3.5-mm hole is drilled through the femur and the first Schanz screw is inserted. The second Schanz screw is introduced into the distal main fragment, as parallel as possible to the first. However, before the hole for the second Schanz screw is drilled, rotation should be checked and any poor alignment of the femur corrected. At least six adjustable clamps are slipped onto each of two long tubes, which are then fixed to both the proximal and the distal Schanz screw.

After reduction of the fracture the remaining four pins are inserted, as far apart from one another as possible. Just as in the tibia, the Schanz screws may be introduced only with the hand chuck, not with the power drill.

Application of axial compression depends upon the fracture pattern or the type of pseudoarthrosis. If, however, there is a *defect* or a comminuted area (Figs. 34–36) no axial compression is possible, but preloading of the Schanz screws is essential to prevent micromovement and thus bone resorption and loosening. Under these circumstances, the Schanz screws are bent away from each other using the adjustable clamps on the inner tube, fixed solidly to it as a turning point (fulcrum). This results in a very strong compression preload between the Schanz screws (see Figs. 36e and 38). As mentioned earlier, placement of the innermost screws close to the fracture will considerably increase stability but may jeopardize a second-step procedure such as plating or nailing.

If *bone contact* at the fracture site is good (transverse or short oblique fracture) axial compression may be very effectively instituted in the following way (Fig. 37a–b): The two innermost adjustable clamps on the inner tube are used as a fulcrum by fixing them solidly and under compression to the tube, but leaving rotational movements "open." By applying distraction to the two corresponding Schanz screws the fracture underneath is also compressed at the opposite cortex, while the adjustable clamps on the outer tube are pushed apart (Fig. 37c). After the two innermost screws have been secured to both tubes, the same procedure is done with the pair of outermost Schanz screws. Finally, the middle pair may be "preloaded" in either direction.

It should be stressed that the stability of the assembly can be considerably improved:

1. By increasing the number of Schanz screws
2. By increasing the distance between the screws
3. By reducing the distance between the tubes and the bone
4. By preloading the Schanz screws against one another in each fragment (Figs. 36e and 38)

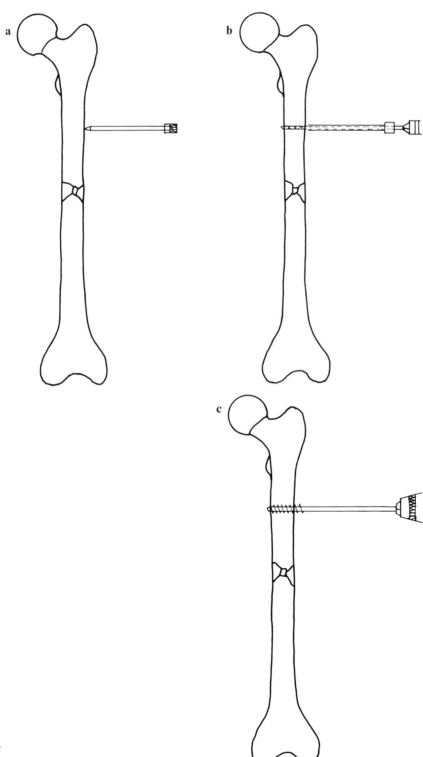

Fig.
34 a–c

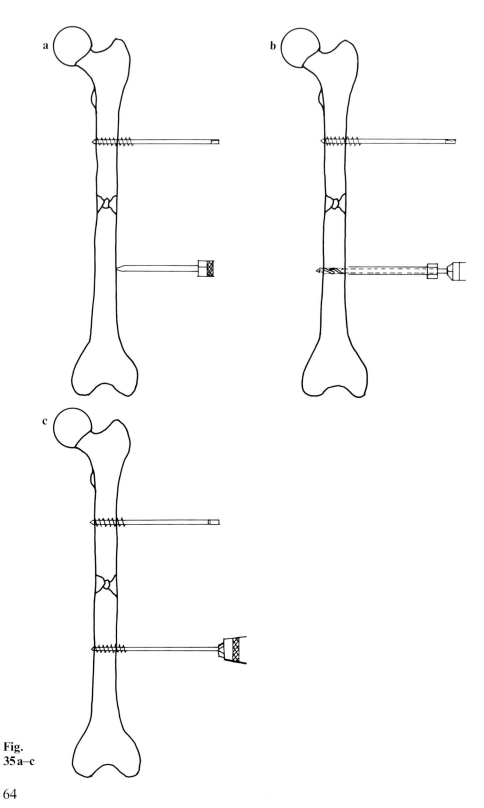

**Fig.
35 a–c**

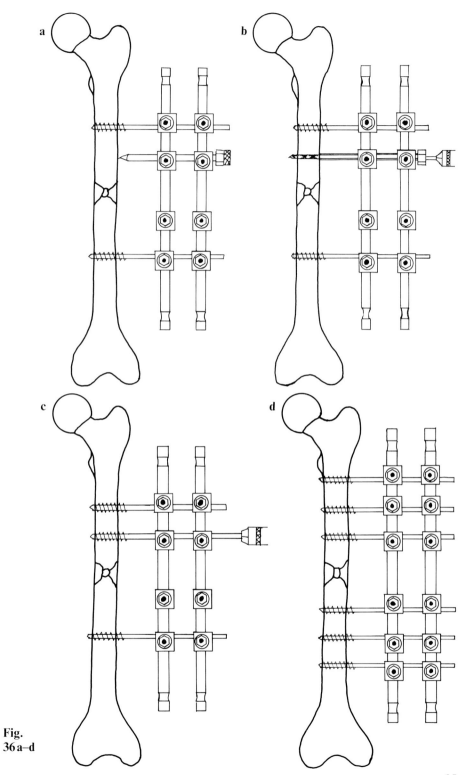

**Fig.
36 a–d**

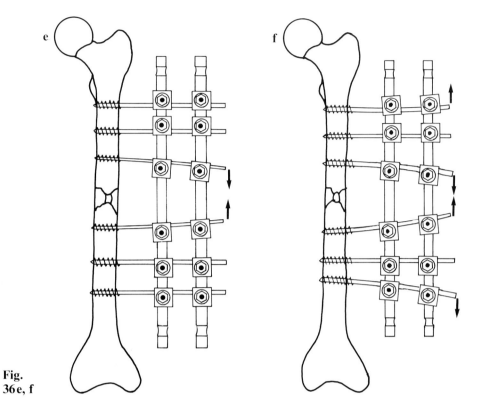

Fig. 36 e, f

66

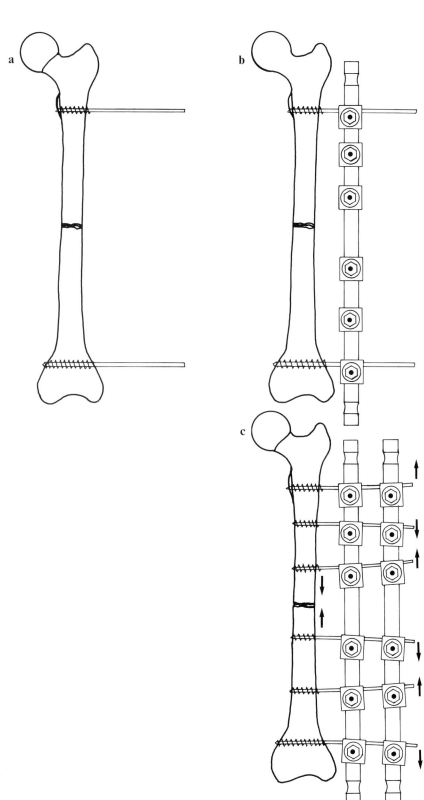

**Fig.
37 a–c**

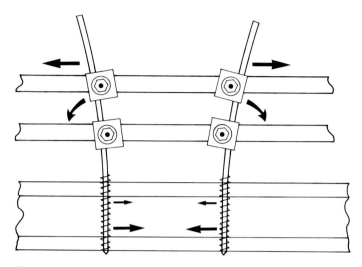

Fig. 38 How to institute preload on Schanz screws within the same fragment to prevent loosening

8 Clinical Application of External Skeletal Fixator

Organizational Prerequisites, Planning, and Preparation of an Operation

External skeletal fixation requires the same preparations as internal fixation or any other surgical procedure. Thus, asepsis must be strictly observed under all circumstances. In draping the extremity, enough points of orientation must be left exposed to permit the evaluation of accurate reduction, particularly in regard to rotation.

Careful preoperative planning is a must in order to decide whether external stabilization will be used only temporarily, or whether it is to be the definitive method of fracture care. Temporary stabilization with the external fixator should be considered mainly in cases of open fractures. Once soft tissue healing and revascularization of the fragments have taken place (usually after 6–8 weeks) internal fixation may be considered, should it prove necessary. If such a later conversion is planned, the Steinmann pins and Schanz screws must be placed as far away from the fracture as possible, which may mean a considerable loss of stability. The preoperative plan must also take into account whether the adjacent joint should temporarily be bridged or not. This will depend, of course, on the nature of the fractures, as well as on the type and degree of soft tissue damage. The unilateral single-plane external fixator provides sufficient stability for this type of temporary immobilization.

In the treatment of fresh open fractures anatomical reduction should generally be carried out before the external fixator is applied. Quite frequently, an interfragmentary lag screw will be able to hold this reduction. We feel that it does not make sense to construct a complex external fixator assembly and only then attempt the reduction of the fracture.

While fresh fractures may be stabilized by temporary unilateral frames, an infected nonunion demands the most stable external fixator assembly. To achieve this high degree of stability, yet at the same time bridge a long segment, the triangular configura-

69

tion appears to be the best method (see pp. 10, 40–44, and 59, 60). In each main fragment one Steinmann pin and/or one Schanz screw is placed as close to the focus of inflammation as is clinically feasible. Of course, the biomechanical rules which govern the relationship of the Schanz screw and the Steinmann pin to bone (axis of rotation and preload) must be kept in mind.

Conversion to Other Forms of Fixation

It mut be stressed that whenever external skeletal fixation is used in diaphyseal fractures one runs the risk of delayed bone healing. Careful and individual evaluation of every fracture is needed in order to decide on the option of any possible further treatment, such as cast bracing, internal fixation, bone grafting, or a combination of the three.

If there is bone loss or extensive comminution such as to preclude any secondary internal fixation, bone grafting should be undertaken early. Secondary bone grafting should also be performed in cases of severe soft tissue injury which renders the conversion to internal fixation almost impossible.

If, on the other hand, the configuration of the fracture and of the wound is such that secondary internal fixation may be considered, X-ray evaluation 6–8 weeks after injury will demonstrate any callus formation or bone healing. If callus formation is encountered, conversion to a weight-bearing brace or to internal fixation is indicated.

A conversion to internal fixation is possible only if the area which will contain the internal fixator was not heavily involved as an anchoring zone for the external skeletal fixator pins and if no pin tract infection is present. Most of the time, therefore, we remove the external fixator before conversion, immobilize the limb for 1–2 weeks in a cast, and carry out internal fixation only when all the points of exit are clean and covered with granulation tissue. Whenever internal fixation is done, a bone graft is recommended as well.

In the treatment of osteitis with instability the external fixator may bring about healing of the infection but not necessarily bony union. If months have passed, if all signs of inflammation and sepsis have disappeared, and if – despite cancellous bone grafting – no bony union is evident, then a conversion of the external skeletal fixation to internal fixation must be considered.

Postoperative Care

The usual rules of postoperative wound care apply; however, some details require emphasis. The wound must be examined every day. Traumatic wounds should be left open whenever possible. Any degree of skin tension at the points of exit of the Steinmann pins or Schanz screws must be avoided. Tension means local ischemia, which frequently leads to sepsis. The exit points should be cleansed regularly. The external fixator permits suspension of the extremity, thus avoiding undesirable pressure on the soft tissues. Most often, early movement of the adjacent joints is possible – except, of course, if the external fixator is bridging an adjacent joint.

The optional removable foot plate prevents postoperative equinus. Once the soft tissues have recovered, further treatment may be ambulatory.

With regard to weight bearing, no fixed schedule can be given. This must be determined individually, and is based on clinical and radiological findings, as well as on the cooperation of the patient. Usually, partial weight bearing (10–15 kg) may be started within 3–4 weeks after injury. We progress to full weight bearing gradually, according to the degree of bony consolidation.

If no conversion to another form of treatment is planned, the rigidity of the external fixator assembly may gradually be reduced by removing parts of the construction, which in turn may enhance bone healing or callus formation. No anesthesia is necessary, but the exit points of the pins and screws must be carefully cleaned and disinfected.

Radiological Examination and Evaluation of Bony Union

Whenever X-rays are ordered the bars of the external fixator must be considered, as they frequently obscure the underlying bone. We feel that two oblique projections are better than the standard AP and lateral; the oblique projections usually give a clear projection of the bone without the overlying metal of the external fixator.

9 Appendix: Special Indications for the Tubular External Fixator

Osteotomy of the Tibial Head and Fixation by Means of the Tubular Fixator

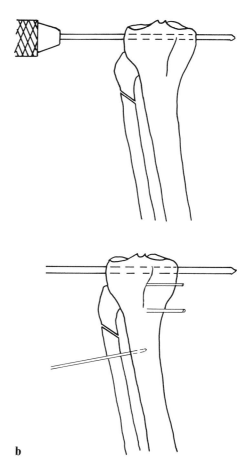

b

Fig. 39   **a** After osteotomy of the fibula, one Steinmann pin is inserted in the frontal plane across the tibial head, about 1.5 cm distal to the joint surface and parallel to it. **b** The osteotomy plane is then marked by means of a Kirschner wire, also in the frontal plane and distal to the planned osteotomy. To control rotation two Kirschner wires are inserted, proximal and distal to the osteotomy in a sagittal plane

Osteotomy of the Tibial Head and Fixation by Means of the Tubular Fixator

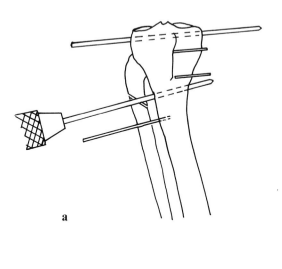

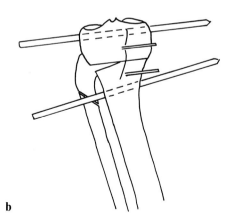

Fig. 40 **a** Insertion of a Steinmann pin in the frontal plane, parallel to the osteotomy-marking Kirschner wire. **b** Osteotomy and removal of a wedge according to the preoperative drawing

Osteotomy of the Tibial Head and Fixation by Means of the Tubular Fixator

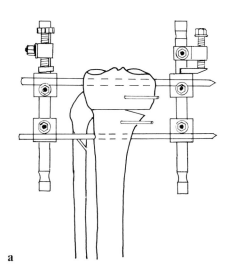

a

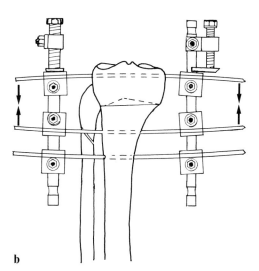

b

Fig. 41 **a** Reduction, application of the tubes with adjustable clamps, and induction of axial compression by means of the compressor or a Verbrugge clamp, or by hand. **b** Fixation of the adjustable clamps once stability is achieved; an additional distal Steinmann pin will increase stability

Osteotomy at the Distal Tibial End and Fixation by Means of the Tubular Fixator

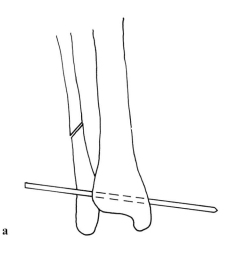

a

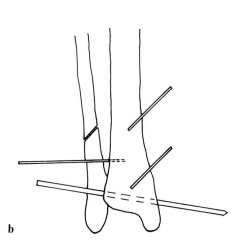

b

Fig. 42a, b Osteotomy of the fibula. **a** Insertion of a Steinmann pin according to the usual procedure, 2 cm proximal to the distal joint and parallel to it. **b** Marking of the correction angle by means of a Kirschner wire in the frontal plane and insertion of two sagittal Kirschner wires to control rotation during osteotomy and fixation

Osteotomy at the Distal Tibial End and Fixation by Means of the Tubular Fixator

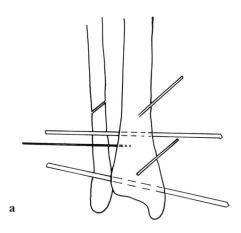

a

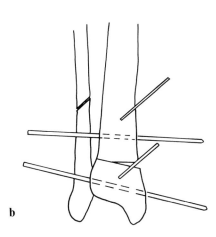

b

Fig. 43 **a** Insertion of the second Steinmann pin in the frontal plane parallel to the marking Kirschner wire, according to the preoperatively determined correction angle. **b** Osteotomy and removal of the wedge as determined in the preoperative planning

Osteotomy at the Distal Tibial End and Fixation by Means of the Tubular Fixator

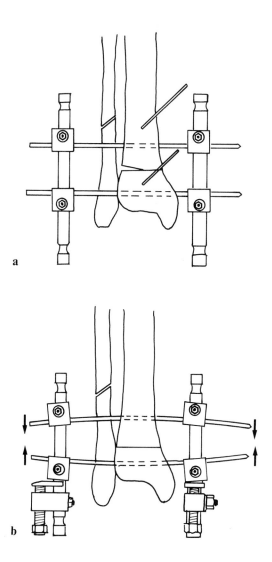

Fig. 44 **a** Reduction and application of the tubes provided with adjustable clamps.
b Institution of axial compression, fixation of the clamps

Arthrodesis of the Knee by Means of the Tubular Fixator

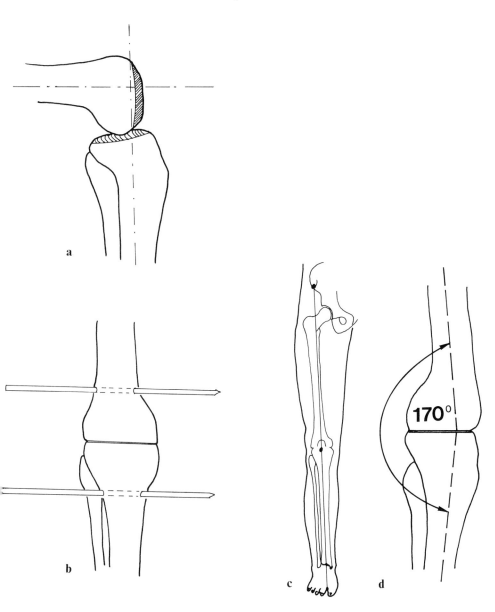

Fig. 45 **a** Resection of the joint cartilage, preserving a slight convexity at the femoral end and a slight concavity at the tibial surface. **b** Reduction in the desired position of the arthrodesis and insertion of Steinmann pins in the frontal plane, in the supracondylar region of the femur and in the tibial head, the pins being parallel to the surface of the arthrodesis. **c, d** Flexion and valgus of about 5°–10° each is recommended for the position of the arthrodesis once reduced

Arthrodesis of the Knee by Means of the Tubular Fixator

The fixation as such shown in Fig. 46 is usually inadequate to secure prompt healing; therefore, one of two methods for achieving additional stability should be selected.

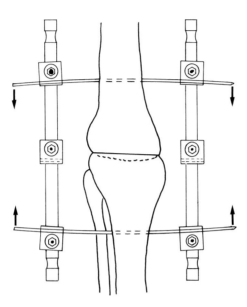

Fig. 46 Application of the tubes with adjustable clamps, and institution of axial compression by approximating the Steinmann pins and fixing the adjustable clamps

Fig. 47 a, b *First possibility*: Transformation of the bilateral frame into a three-dimensional frame. Proximal and distal to the arthrodesis surface a Schanz screw is inserted into the sagittal plane. The sagittal Schanz screws, united by a tube, are connected to the bilateral frame by means of Steinmann pins. Preloading these two screws by compressing them against each other is recommended. This ventral tube has a very effective tension-band action

Arthrodesis of the Knee by Means of the Tubular Fixator

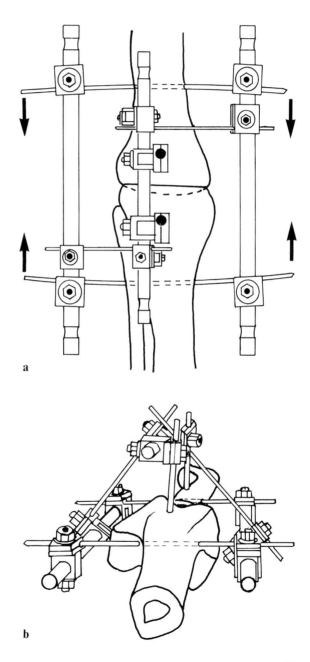

a

b

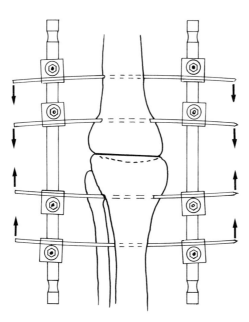

Fig. 48 The *second possibility* consists in adding a Steinmann pin on each side of the arthrodesis, in the same plane as the first two Steinmann pins. To insert the second pair of Steinmann pins, the aiming device is very useful (see p. 27). The technique is explained in detail, using the distal tibia as an example (see p. 54, Fig. 29i, j). The additional Steinmann pins are also preloaded as shown.

Arthrodesis of the Tibiotarsal Joint by Means of the Tubular Fixator

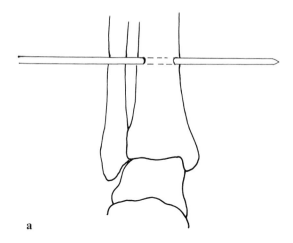

a

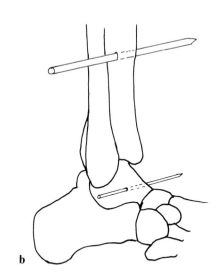

b

Fig. 49   **a** About 6 cm above the tibiotarsal joint a Steinmann pin is inserted into the tibia in a frontal plane. **b** A Kirschner wire parallel to the Steinmann pin is inserted in the neck of the talus

Arthrodesis of the Tibiotarsal Joint by Means of the Tubular Fixator

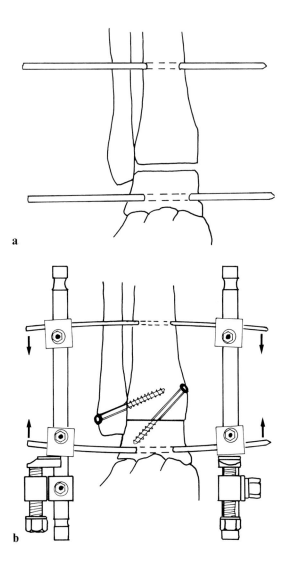

Fig. 50 **a** After chiseling off of the joint surfaces of tibia, talus, and malleolus, the Kirschner wire in the neck of the talus is replaced by a Steinmann pin. **b** Reduction to the desired position of the arthrodesis and addition of tubes with adjustable clamps to institute compression along the tube; the compression effect is counteracted by the Achilles tendon, which functions as a tension band. Additional lag screw fixation of the denuded fibula and between tibia and talus adds to the stability of the arthrodesis

Addendum

Coauthor: FRIDOLIN SÉQUIN, Dipl. Ing. ETH

Since completion of the manual some additional findings have significantly added to the armamentarium of external fixation.

1. It has been found that *Schanz screws provided with short threads*, which anchor in the far cortex only, offer several advantages:

   – A Schanz screw with a short thread (18 mm) crossing the near cortex as a solid bar offers much greater stiffness than a Schanz screw with a long thread in both cortices, as its stiffness corresponds to the diameter of the shaft and not to that of the core of the thread. It can be shown that 4.5-mm Schanz screws with short threads anchoring only in the far cortex give an even more rigid system than 5.0-mm Schanz screws with long threads (Fig. A 1 a–c).
   – Providing the Schanz screws with a short thread permits the use of the same kind of screws regardless of the bone diameter, and it is only necessary to have a sufficient variety of overall lengths (Fig. A 1 d).
   – The unilateral frame gains considerably more bending stability and some more torsional stability if two bars in close proximity to each other are connected to the Schanz screws (Fig. A 2).
   – The 4.5-mm Schanz screw permits the use of the standard 3.5/4.5-mm instruments when preparing the holes for the screws.

2. To facilitate insertion of Schanz screws, new *drill sleeves with an inner diameter of 5 mm* (outer diameter 6 mm) corresponding with the existing 3.5-mm sleeves and trocars have been added (Fig. A 3).
   Drilling of 3.5-mm and 4.5-mm holes and insertion of the Schanz screws can be done across these sleeves. This greatly facilitates the localization of the drill holes in the bone.

3. The *adjustable clamps* (no. 393.64) are now produced to accept the new drill sleeves with outer diameter of 6 mm (Fig. A 4). Existing clamps can be modified by SYNTHES manufacturers.

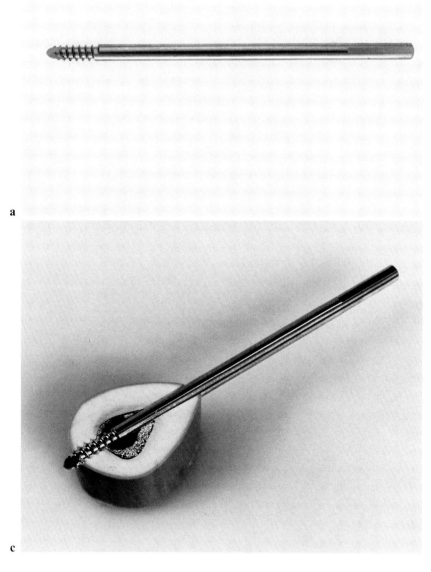

a

c

Fig. A 1 **a** Short-threaded (18-mm) Schanz screw; **b** threaded end; **c** short-threaded Schanz screw anchoring in opposite cortex; **d** available short-threaded Schanz screws

86

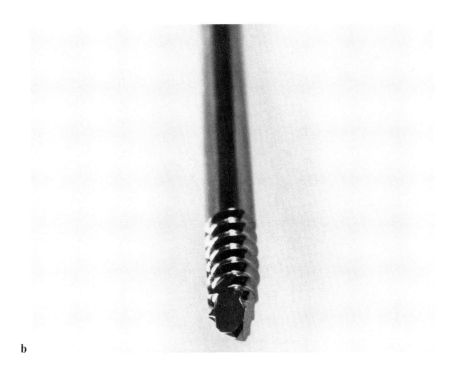

b

L = 100 − 200 mm

d

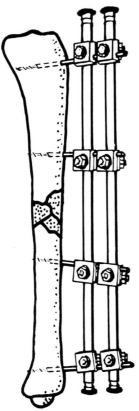

Fig. A2   Double-bar assembly of unilateral frame

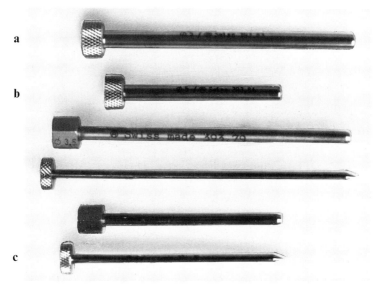

Fig. A3   New 5-mm drill sleeve, long (**a**) and short (**b**), corresponding with (existing) 3.5-mm drill sleeves and trocar (**c**)

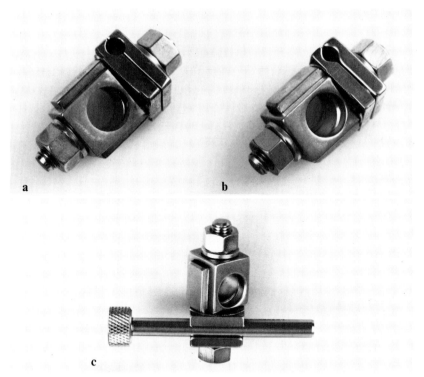

a

b

c

Fig.
A 4

a Old (for diameter up to 5-mm) and **b** new (for diameter up to 6 mm) adjustable clamps. (Old clamps can be modified!) **c** Adjustable clamp with new 5-mm drill sleeve

The four steps for Schanz screw insertion are illustrated in Fig. A 5. They are as follows.

a) Assemble 5-mm and 3.5-mm drill sleeves with 3.5-mm trocar and penetrate through stab incision onto bone surface.
b) Remove trocar and drill with 3.5-mm drill bit through both cortices.
c) Remove 3.5-mm drill sleeve and overdrill near cortex to 4.5 mm.
d) Insert 4.5-mm Schanz screw into bone through remaining 5-mm drill sleeve using universal chuck with handle. Only now remove the 5-mm drill sleeve. The Schanz screw is now ready to accept the adjustable clamps (see the details below of the operative steps of unilateral fixation).

4. In "salvage cases" with no possibility of internal fixation on account of poor – particularly infected – soft tissues, *bilateral*

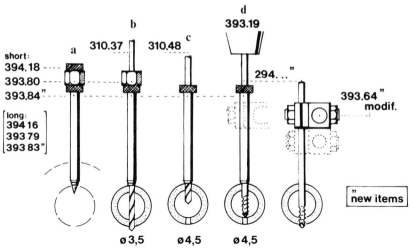

Fig. A5 Operative steps for inserting a short-threaded Schanz screw

or preferably triangular frames should be applied, using Steinmann pins as close to the focus of instability as possible.

For easier insertion and less heat generation, the *Steinmann pins* are now provided with a *modified drill bit point* which has a very obtuse angle and therefore enters the predrilled hole easily and can be left exposed without the risk of hurting the patient or the nursing staff (Fig. A6).

The three steps for insertion of 5-mm Steinmann pins are as follows (Fig. A7):

a) Assemble 5-mm and 3.5-mm drill sleeves with 3.5-mm trocar and penetrate through stab incision onto the bone surface.

b) Remove trocar and 3.5-mm drill sleeve, drill through both cortices with 4.5-mm drill bit.

Important Remark: In constructing a bilateral or triangular frame, the aiming device has to be used. It is inserted through the adjustable clamps. Step **b** is therefore subdivided into two sequences:

– Drill a 3.5-mm hole through the 3.5-mm drill sleeve of the aiming device, which in turn is inserted into the 5-mm drill sleeve.

– Remove the aiming device and overdrill the 3.5-mm hole using the 4.5-mm drill bit through the 5-mm drill sleeve, which has remained place.

90

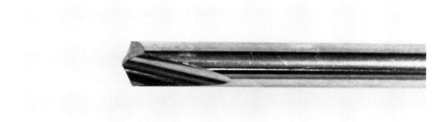

Fig.
A6   Modified drill bit point of Steinmann pin

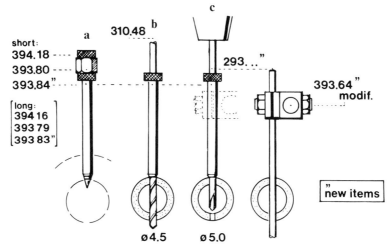

Fig.   Operative steps for inserting Steinmann pin with drill point (see also " Im-
A7   portant Remark " in text)

This maneuver will assure a precise location of the Steinmann
pin with regard to the opposite adjustable clamp.

c) Insert Steinmann pin with universal chuck with handle through
5-mm drill sleeve. The Steinmann pin is now ready to accept
the adjustable clamps.

Single-Bar Unilateral Fixation

Indication: Second-degree and third-degree open fractures with
two main fragments, with or without butterfly fragment.
Principle: Preliminary interfragmentary lag screw fixation plus
neutralization by external fixator.

The operative steps are as follows:

1. Screw fixation (mostly possible through traumatic wound without need for further exposure).
2. Insertion of the most distal Schanz screw (Drill both cortices to 3.5 mm and overdrill near cortex to 4.5 mm).
3. Insertion of the most proximal Schanz screw
4. Application of the tube with four (modified or new) 6-mm adjustable clamps mounted to the tube.
5. This procedure can very often be regarded as definitive. The Schanz screws can therefore be placed to assure maximum stability: screws 3 and 4 are placed close to the fracture, thus permitting a maximum distance between the two screws in each main fragment. For the application of screws 3 and 4 the "drill sleeves-trocar assembly" will be inserted through the new (or modifield old) adjustable clamps.
6. Additional preloading of the Schanz screws, either *inter*fragmentally (across the fracture focus) or preferably *intra*fragmentally, is recommended.

Double-Bar Unilateral Fixation

Indication: Comminuted fractures or fractures with bone loss
Principle: To increase rigidity we use two parallel tubes in close proximity and as close to the bone as possible.

Although fixation with one tube provides surprisingly good stability, *double-bar unilateral fixation* considerably increases stiffness and is therefore recommended. It does not take much more space if one allows minimal distance between the two tubes. Depending on the soft tissue injury, we choose between the strictly sagittal single-plane arrangement and the one coming more from the medial aspect. (To further increase stability, a V-shaped arrangement of two unilateral fixators may be chosen.)

The operative steps are as follows:

1. Insertion of the most distal Schanz screw.
2. Insertion of a Schanz screw as proximally as possible.
3. Simultaneous application of the two tubes provided with four (six) adjustable clamps each. Reduction should be controlled at that moment. Careful attention should be given to the rotation of the distal fragment, using the opposite side as a control.

4. Insertion of the second distal Schanz screw. Placing of this Schanz screw depends on the long-range planning. If a secondary procedure is planned, one should keep away from the fracture focus as much as possible, still keeping the two Schanz screws approximately 5 cm apart. If no internal fixation is anticipated, then the Schanz screw can be placed as close to the fracture as possible to gain a maximum of stability.
5. Insertion of the second proximal screw. With regard to placing, the same rules apply as in step 4. (For drilling for steps 4 and 5, see step 5 of the procedure for single-bar unilateral fixation.)
6. *Intra*fragmental preload should be applied (according to Fig. 38 in the manual).

Recapitulation Concerning Preload of Steinmann Pins and Schanz-Screws

Any implant under weight-bearing stress which is not preloaded against its site in the bone will undergo micromovements and thus induce bone resorption, which in turn leads to loosening of the implant. There are various ways to achieve the desired preload when using external fixation in connection with Steinmann pins or Schanz screws.

1. *Steinmann pins* used in a bilateral or triangular frame can be easily preloaded against each other by slight bending. This will usually need to be done within the same fragment (*intra*-fragmental preload), but if adequate lag screw fixation of the fracture is possible, then axial (*inter*fragmental) preload can be instituted. It should be remembered that any tension on the skin caused by the pins should be released by a short incision.
2. Two *Schanz screws* can easily be put under additional preload *intra*fragmentally by bending them against each other. This is possible when using one tube only, but much easier when two parallel tubes are used (Fig. 38 in the manual).

Double-bar application with six Schanz screws is essential in the femur.
Preloading across the fracture plane with *inter*fragmentary compression in the absence of lag screws is very difficult to achieve and is not recommended because of the kinking effect exerted on the fracture focus.

References

1 Anderson R (1936) An ambulatory method of treating fractures of the shaft of the femur. Surg Gynecol Obst 62:865
2 Behrens F, Searls K (1982) Unilateral external fixation experience with the ASIF "tubular" frame. In: Uhthoff HK (ed) Current concepts of external fixation of fractures. Springer, Berlin Heidelberg New York
2a Claudi B, Rittmann WW, Rüedi T (1976) Anwendung des Fixateur externe bei der Primärversorgung offener Frakturen. Helv Chir Acta 4:469–471
3 Codivilla A (1904) Means of lengthening in lower limbs the muscles and tissues which are shortened through deformity. A J Orth Surg 3:353
4 Hax PM (1984) Mechanische Untersuchungen zum Klammerfixateur externe. Dissertation, Gesamthochschule Essen (in press)
5 Hierholzer G, Kleining R, Hörster G, Zemenides P (1978) External fixation. Classification and indications. Arch Orthop Trauma Surg 92:175
6 Hoffmann R (1942) Percutane Frakturbehandlung. Chirurg 14:101
7 Kleining R (1981) Der Fixateur externe an der Tibia. Hefte Unfallheilkd 151: (monograph)
8 Kleining R, Chernowitz A (1982) The stability of different systems. A comparative study. In: Uhthoff HK (ed) Current concepts of external fixation of fractures. Springer, Berlin Heidelberg New York
9 Kleining R, Hierholzer G (1976) Biomechanische Untersuchung zur Osteosynthese mit dem Fixateur externe. Acta Trauma 6:71
10 Lambotte A (1908) Sur l'osteosynthèse. Belg Med 231
11 Malgaigne JF (1853) Considèrations cliniques sur les fractures de la rotule et leur traitment par les griffes. J des Connaissances Med Pratiques 16:9
12 Müller KH (1982) Therapy of post-traumatic osteomyelitis. In: Uhthoff HK (ed) Current concepts of external fixation of fractures. Springer, Berlin Heidelberg New York
13 Müller ME (1955) Die Kompressionsosteosynthese unter besonderer Berücksichtigung der Kniearthrodese. Helv Chir Acta 6:474
14 Müller ME, Allgöwer M, Willenegger H (1977) Manual der Osteosynthese. Springer, Berlin Heidelberg New York
15 Niederer PG, Chiquet C (1980) Mechanical principles of external fixation, with particular consideration of stability. Internatl. Fixateur externe Symposion, Duisburg. AO International, Berne
16 Stader O (1939) Treating fractures of long bones with the reduction splint. North Am Vet 20:55
17 Vidal J, Rabischong P, Bonnel F, Adrey J (1970) Etude biomèchanique du fixateur externe d'Hoffmann dans les fractures de jambe. Montpellier Chir 16:43

18 Weller S (1982) The external fixator for the prevention and treatment of infections. In: Uhthoff HK (ed) Current concepts of external fixation of fractures. Springer, Berlin Heidelberg New York

Subject Index

T. Rüedi, A. H. C. v. Hochstetter, R. Schlumpf

Surgical Approaches for Internal Fixation

Translated from the German by T. C. Telger
Foreword by M. Allgöwer
1984. 99 figures, partly in color. IX, 187 pages.
ISBN 3-540-12809-3

Manual of Internal Fixation

Techniques Recommended by the AO Group

by **M. E. Müller, M. Allgöwer, R. Schneider, H. Willenegger**
In collaboration with numerous experts
Translated from the German by J. Schatzker
2nd expanded and revised edition. 1979. 345 figures in
colour, 2 Templates for Preoperative Planning.
X, 409 pages. ISBN 3-540-09227-7

C. F. Brunner, B. G. Weber

Special Techniques in Internal Fixation

Translated from the German by T. C. Telger
1982. 91 figures. X, 198 pages. ISBN 3-540-11056-9

U. Heim, K. M. Pfeiffer

Small Fragment Set Manual

Technique Recommended by the ASIF Group

Translated from the German by R. L. Batten, K. M. Pfeiffer
2nd revised and enlarged edition. 1982. 215 figures in more
than 500 separate illustrations. IX, 396 pages.
ISBN 3-540-11143-3

F. Séquin, R. Texhammar

AO/ASIF Instrumentation

Manual of Use and Care

Introduction and Scientific Aspects by H. Willenegger
Translated from the German by T. C. Telger
1981. Approx. 1300 figures, 17 separate Checklists.
XVI, 306 pages. ISBN 3-540-10337-6

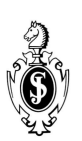

Springer-Verlag
Berlin
Heidelberg
New York
Tokyo

Springer AV
Instruction Programme

Films/Videocassettes:

Theoretical and practical bases of internal fixation, results of experimental research:
Internal Fixation – Basic Principles and Modern Means
The Biomechanics of Internal Fixation
The Ligaments of the Knee Joint. Pathophysiology

Internal fixation of fractures and reconstructive bone surgery:
Interal Fixation of Forearm Fractures
Internal Fixation of Noninfected Diaphyseal Pseudarthroses
Internal Fixation of Malleolar Fractures
Internal Fixation of Patella Fractures
Medullary Nailing
Internal Fixation of the Distal End of the Humerus
Internal Fixation of Mandibular Fractures
Corrective Osteotomy of the Distal Tibia
Internal Fixation of Tibial Head Fractures (available in German only)

Joint replacement:
Total Hip Prostheses (3 parts)
Part 1: Instruments, Operation on Model
Part 2: Operative Technique
Part 3: Complications. Special Cases
Elbow-Arthroplasty with the New GSB-Prosthesis
Total Wrist Joint Replacement

Replantation surgery:
Microsurgery for Accidents

Slide Series:

ASIF-Technique for Internal Fixation of Fractures
Manual of Internal Fixation
Small Fragment Set Manual
Internal Fixation of Patella and Malleolar Fractures
Total Hip Prosteses
Operation on Model and in vivo, Complications and Special Cases

● Please ask for information material
● Order from:
Springer-Verlag Heidelberger Platz 3, D-1000 Berlin 33, or
Springer-Verlag New York Inc., 175 Fifth Avenue,
New York, Ny 10010, USA

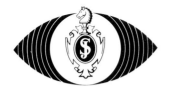

Springer-Verlag
Berlin
Heidelberg
New York
Tokyo